Retirement:

Sacred or Scared

Retirement:

Sacred or Scared

Nancy Lee Burns

Nancy Lee Burns

ISBN: 978-0-9815814-4-6
Library of Congress Control Number: 2009932054

Written by Nancy Lee Burns
Edited and produced by Pamela R. Goodfellow
Cover illustration: Donald Jenny
Book Design: The Printed Page

Dedication

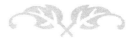

In honor of the movie "The Bucket List" and Betty.

Special thanks to Dr. Michelle Medrano,
New Vision Spiritual Growth Center, Scottsdale, Arizona

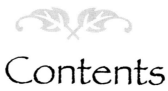

Contents

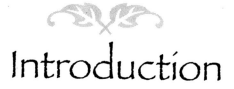

Introduction

Forty some years ago I volunteered as a candy stripe girl in the hospital wing of a Catholic home for old folks. A disgruntled patient in a tiny room at the end of the hall was identified as a "problem patient" because she had anger issues and refused to communicate. I, being an eager candy stripe volunteer, wanted to please people, and raised my hand to volunteer to help this patient.

"I'll do it, she can't be any worse than some of the old timers in my family." Many adults in my world drank, got angry, and became irrational. As a child I learned to walk on eggshells and became invisible. The patient became my assignment; I had no competition. The first time I entered her room it was with a little trepidation. My first impression was shock. My eyes surveyed this huge sleeping mass in her bed with blankets piled and pulled up around her chin. I moved closer. Her face appeared blotchy, probably age spots. What struck me most was this flowering, flowing mop of red and grey hair that surrounded her blotchy face like a halo. Against the white pillowcases her hair looked like a huge red bush with grey flowers growing from under the covers. It was long, thick and medusa-like in its movement as she took deep breaths. I stared in amazement that a human being was buried under all those blankets and hair. She was bedridden and very old.

I pulled a chair next to the bed and watched her chest heave up and down as she slept. This was going to be easy. Boredom began to creep in and I, being a high school student, realized how slowly time goes by just sitting in a chair listening to someone snore. My eyes looked around the room, which was full of color. The rug was splashed with red and green designs and very old, probably what I would now call a Persian rug. The ceiling lamp I decided was institutional but I wondered who hung the blue paper butterflies from it. The dresser with its white lace cover was full of pictures of family. Fresh flowers adorned her night stand and some stuffed animals sat in folding chairs staring back at me. There in the corner tucked under an old brass lamp with a frilly shade was an old phonograph player. I could just imagine the old dog from the RCA commercials coming out to listen with its head and ears tilted as though listening intently. Very quietly I got up and tiptoed over to the old forty-five record player in the corner. Timidly I clicked it on. Carefully I placed the needle arm in the groove on the forty-five record and made sure the volume was very low. First I heard crackling and then the song *He Danced with the Girl with the Strawberry Curls and the Band Played on.*

The music played softly so I sat back down and underneath my breath began to hum. The mass under the bed covers, whose name I learned from staff was Betty, rustled and opened her eyes. Her blue eyes blazed through me. She grumbled.

"I don't like humming, sing for God's sake, you fool, sing if you are going to open your mouth."

My fear barometer deep inside my stomach skyrocketed like I was going to throw up. Now I was busted, this woman who didn't talk was telling me what to do. The fear tripped my rebellious teenager self into action and I wanted to strike back, but didn't.

I was thinking, no way old lady. Maybe it was a typical teenager reaction. This lady, Betty, who didn't even know me, couldn't tell me what to do. Then I rationalized; after all, I was sitting in her room and she hadn't met me either. So I moved into my critical self. Let me judge me before she judged me. So I opened my mouth.

"I don't sing." Both of her piercing eyes were wide open as her voice exploded in a rusty high pitch squeak.

"Everyone sings. Open your mouth to form words and let the humming come out."

I swear Betty analyzed all my fears, but specifically my fear of singing. Maybe it was her blue eyes but there was sensitivity in the way she focused on me. I wasn't invisible to her. She paid attention to me. So I figured she must be wise. In retrospect I was sure my blue eyes were startlingly open like a deer in headlights. Betty stared me down.

"Be true to yourself and don't give a damn about what others think, sing, and sing from your heart. Every one can sing!"

Her smile made me feel safe in her presence. I had no idea what my expression was in the moment but I knew and she knew we had a bond. We understood each other. It was like when you wave an unspoken hi to someone and they wave back. No words are exchanged but you know you have been noticed. I couldn't bluff her. She saw me. We both began singing louder and louder until a shocked nun came in and closed the door. Betty looked at me.

"Sing louder, child." We did and the nun came back.

"Keep it down."

We did. I got in trouble because Betty and I made too much noise. It was so fun to break the rules and sing with an old lady.

Betty didn't care because she was laughing too. It was a life lesson because I broke through an old taboo of nuns being in charge. Betty was in charge of her room. We weren't hurting anyone and our singing wasn't that bad. In that afternoon I learned to sing anyway. Betty didn't care if we were loud or off key. I learned not to be so concerned about what others thought. Sing anyway. When we both stopped laughing I poured us some water. She told me about her husband and how they met. He was deceased but her smile got even wider and her eyes watered as she asked me to bring his picture from the dresser to the bed. Betty's hair had been bright red since birth I learned and her husband loved the thickness and the color of her hair. It was what drew him to her. They loved to dance and their song was *He Danced with the Girl with the Strawberry Curls and the Band Played on.* I was excited to hear about her wedding and her past. I danced over to the record player and played "their song" again. Betty held her husband's picture close to her heart and fell back asleep. Hearing her story made me feel like her friend, after all, she was my first married friend telling me about her husband. She trusted me to tell me about her life.

We visited many times together. She loved me and was the grandmother I never knew. Whatever silly thing happened to me in school or at home, she was interested in it. I felt welcomed in her room perhaps more than I had felt anywhere at the time. I was a teenager and other adults were too busy to listen to me. If she could have, she would have baked cookies for me. So I bought, and brought, bakery cookies to her. She didn't care they weren't homemade. To this day I give store-bought cookies and feel good about it. Forty years later I wondered why she was never difficult and uncommunicative with me. At the time no one asked me and I never gave it a second thought. Now I know the answer, we sang together. She knew I was real and always made me sing loud every visit so my heart could hear.

"Your heart is more important than your ears," she would say. In retrospect Betty taught me perception; how to look at things, especially with my heart. And also the power of breaking though fears.

"Just sing dear."

One day I went to her room and it was empty. She had passed away and no one thought to inform me. I was just a teenage candy stripe volunteer. The staff's dislike for Betty probably rippled into dislike for me. Not notifying me of her death validated within me the message; I don't matter, I don't count. I felt numb. I smiled thinking of Betty happy in heaven dancing with her husband. If I could have, I would have played the old record player but the room was bare. I waited until I got home to cry. Sadness must have covered my face because they sent me home early.

"No work for you today."

In retrospect I became visible in Betty's eyes. She sowed seeds in my psyche that are still unfolding even some after forty years of laying dormant.

"I don't like humming, sing for God's sake, you fool, sing if you are going to open your mouth, everyone sings. Open your mouth to form words and let the humming come out. Be true to yourself and don't give a damn about what others think, sing, sing from your heart. Every one can sing!"

Retirement: Am I Scared or Am I Sacred?

Section I:
Journal Entries

October 1
The Key—Sacred or Scared

It usually began as I watched someone retire. Questions and visions of what retirement would look like for me occupied my mind. I wanted to know the answer of what to do in retirement. As others retired I wondered if my day would ever come. Finally that day happened.

Some, I learned associated retirement with death. Some had a retirement party and started a new job the following week. I knew there were lots of things to do when I retired. Pre-retirement was a space of postponed dreams and provided an excuse as to why my dreams weren't fulfilled. My mind did not accept "my dreams would never happen" so I piled all my dreams on a back burner. Stalling and saying later to my dreams was a form of denial. It struck me as similar to putting money in the bank for some future date. Bury my acorns or save for a rainy day. I saved my dreams for when I had time rather than make time for them. Work and dreams were mutually exclusive unless I counted being self-sufficient as a dream. I don't remember exactly when being self-sufficient shifted from being a dream to a driving force that overshadowed my dreams. Be that as it may, it happened.

I remember age five associated with kindergarten; age seven with First Holy Communion; age sixteen with driving; age eighteen with three/two beer or the military draft; and age twenty-one with voting. My only thought regarding a future age after twenty-one was turning sixty-five. My dad was forced to retire at age sixty-five and here I was retiring at age fifty-five. I remembered being so excited to drive at age sixteen. Maybe the next exciting age after turning twenty-one would be turning sixty-five and retiring. Marriages and births weren't associated with a particular age and were milestones but not milestone ages like sixteen, eighteen, etc. I thought it would be a big deal to retire but to retire early at age fifty-five became a nice exclamation point. The only age between twenty-one and sixty-five I celebrated to date was age thirty. It was an Irish wake with wailers who mourned my youth and welcomed my adulthood. At the time I never gave a thought to turning sixty-five or even retiring. It was too far down the road. At age sixty-two when I collect social security, if it is still here, I will celebrate.

Sometime in my late forties I heard others at work proclaim; "I only have three years to retirement" or "Six months to retirement." I became painfully aware that the time left until retirement sounded like time left to complete a prison sentence. Six months and somebody got out. It wasn't as if anyone said, "Six months and I get to stay longer." No one I knew was forced to retire or get out. I wanted out. Thoughts of my retirement began percolating in my brain. Make no mistake I wasn't a prisoner; I wanted to get to the finish line and then go dig up all those buried acorns.

I remember the year when I turned fifty-four and finally, finally, became eligible to retire. My employer had a rule of eighty. When age plus service years equaled eighty, retirement became an option. Fifty-four and a half years of age added to my twenty-six years of work time passed the eighty mark. My pension was based on years of service times two. Twenty-five years of service times two equaled fifty percent of my salary. Evaluating my future budgets and trimming my lifestyle gave me the green light to retire.

My thoughts prior to retiring centered around wow I could be free of the nine to seven routine or whatever cute analogy I thought of in the moment. It was fairly frightening. Being a good little workaholic, work was my life. Now I began to think about replacing the work model with a freedom model. Here I was working since I was sixteen and now at age fifty-four my thoughts were on retirement. The fear was I could make a mistake and be unable to live on fifty percent of my salary. I had no fears of unoccupied time. I knew I had a huge storage vault in my brain of things I wanted to do. Other people I knew had retired before me. I got personal with them and asked questions about finances. My research discovered their expenditures were less than estimated. One person reversed his decision to draw six hundred dollars a month from his IRA to his pension. He discovered his pension was enough. One person out of the ten had a negative experience. His health insurance increased dramatically for him and his wife. He had returned to work to foot his insurance bill. .

My mind was mysterious. As the decision to retire swirled I experienced full throttle the impulse to leave but with one stipulation. My goals needed to be completed and finished well. I knew successful completion was optimal. It was clear what I was leaving but what I would do in the future was unclear. I focused one hundred percent on leaving my career in good stead. It was the power of choice that moved me forward. Many friends suggested I leave work at the moment of eligibility and others suggested staying until age sixty-two or sixty-five. The bottom line was only I knew the best time to exit work. It turned out to be age fifty-five and it was perfect. It was similar to a million dollar lottery win. I became financially independent. I honored everyone in his or her respective space and was full of gratitude to have learned so much about compassion. It was easy to have compassion for those I had loved and honored. True compassion however involves love for all sentient beings, which included the liars and thieves. The liars and thieves were human beings who made mistakes and needed compassion, not excuses. Lies were confronted and mandatory to confront in my communication. Those who stayed stuck in the lies made that choice and suffered consequences. That was when I learned compassion. I had no control over another's ethics or denial. I looked them in the eye and knew. They were human beings, like me, who had made mistakes along the way. There was no condoning just compassion.

Another old phrase that popped up in my psyche was "love your enemy." Within my own consciousness I healed many parts of myself. The liar and thief lived in me also. Needing to lie to please another was a lesson. It was easier to see it in others than in myself. Nothing anyone said stopped me in my own denials and lies, it was an inside job. The mirror of life looked back at me as I gazed into it. I learned to forgive the liars and thieves who taught me to better understand those parts of myself that lie and steal. This birthed compassion. Without those people on my path I would have stayed in judgment and thought I was so much better. They are as human as am I.

The key to retirement for me was a suitable pension. Overnight I became financially and emotionally free to explore the universe. Financial freedom was not a birthright. I had the Midwestern work ethic. I was taught the only time one could call in sick to work was for death or a serious disease. Here I was at age fifty-five with signed retirement paperwork. Sometimes a person outgrows his place of employment and I did. Everyone has heard "you can't beat city hall." There is a culture in every organization and I outgrew it. It spit me out like a leaf in a tornado. In my mind I confronted what needed to be confronted and moved on. I learned to do what was right rather than what was easy. In other words staying in my job was less attractive than exploring freedom in retirement. As a workaholic I was addicted to work. I stepped into freedom.

Retirement: Sacred or Scared

The decision to retire became solid but the journey revolved around being sacred or scared. Little did I realize at the time that whichever I focused on, sacred or scared, determined the answer. Whatever I thought, there I was, and it impacted my outcome. Many times my reaction to things was bigger than the thing itself. Being negative created a dark, scary environment. Being depressed brought about an atmosphere of sadness. It was like the bad apple in the batch that permeated the whole bushel. Being happy, joyous and full of laughter created a happier environment. Expectation determined outcome. There were people who predicted death at retirement or said retired people don't know what to do with themselves. Those negative seeds didn't take root in my mind; I chose to become conscious of my own more positive belief systems. I had heard of others and knew a few who did die shortly after retirement but not me. Some found jobs after several months because, as they said, they were bored. It made me examine my own belief systems about retirement. I concluded I was either going to be sacred or scared in the process and I chose.

A workshop I attended many years ago taught me that love and fear are all that exist. There were shades of grey in the love and fear. Sacred meant prayerful, divine, trust. Scared meant fear in all its manifestations. Fear and prayer are mutually exclusive. My thoughts and belief systems translated into being scared or sacred with nothing in between. I likened it to traveling up or down. The direction of my thinking was more important than the speed. Every moment I choose. When I found myself in fear I remembered sacred and turned my being in that direction. A better way of saying it is that sacred and scared are directions more than locations.

I began retirement and subconsciously created a new job description. My self-given assignment was to clean closets stuffed with boxes stored for twenty plus years. My life was written on paper in those boxes. Somewhere in unloading the twentieth box I realized I had replaced my old job description with another one for home. It was not a good idea. Working so many years with a model of doing, doing, doing, moved me automatically to look for something to do. I wanted my retirement to be about being myself not meeting goals. So I began a ceremony that blessed and released all the memories associated with the contents of the boxes. In cleaning I had sown the seed for a huge yard sale. There was a pause at one box of books when I found an old Playboy magazine and wondered about its origin. As an old feminist I knew I didn't buy it. Flipping through the pages I realized it contained the Jimmy Carter interview about lust in his heart that caused so much commotion way back when. Times have changed.

I found old love letters/pictures/journals all taking me back in a time capsule. Long buried feelings erupted, some into sadness and some joy. It was like meeting someone I had forgotten about and knew a long time ago. Only it was I looking at a younger less wise version of myself. Surely all these years later I have learned a lot about myself. My choice in men was pretty good; I just hadn't been ready for commitment. There were lots of forks in the road with choices; if I knew then what I know now I would choose differently. The wiser part of me knew it took mistakes to learn what I know. What I know in the realm of things isn't much but certainly a lot more than I knew as a young woman.

The garage sale included mountain climbing gear, tennis equipment, and lots of old photography books. I kept the old cameras. I shredded mountains of old paper all the while remembering some old poem "one hundred years from now this paperwork won't mean a thing." And it didn't. Enjoying the journey and staying in the sacred moment were what mattered to me.

October 10
Old Dreams—Alive or Buried

I learned dreams buried long ago were still consuming energy. Physically there was a release of energy as I threw away a photo of an old boyfriend. Placing my tennis and mountain climbing gear into the sell pile for my garage sale created a whoosh or a vacuum in my psyche. In the same way these items took up storage space in my garage they took up space and energy in my psyche. I was shocked that my heartbeat skipped at the boyfriend picture lying in the garbage heap. Reading the old love letters brought tears to my eyes and now the letters were scattered about in a garbage can. It had been twenty some years. It was better to experience repressed feelings than keeping them dormant. Had I not saved the items those repressed feelings might still be within me eating up energy. Not being recognized doesn't stop the truth from being the truth. Once the energy left my system fresh new thoughts emerged. And I thought I was just cleaning house. In reality I was cleaning my subconscious. I knew something good would grow because I planted positive seeds in the vacated space. Nature abhorres a vacuum.

It took energy in the beginning to bury feelings and it took energy to keep them buried. Some dreams got thrown away like the old boyfriend's picture and some had to grow up or fast forward. At age four I wanted a tricycle, at six a two wheel bicycle and at sixteen a car. Old dreams like shadows coming to life emerged. Dreams of writing, painting, sculpting, taking pictures, being a mom, and having a family came to light. Climbing Mt. Everest and skiing in Switzerland reawakened as afterthoughts. Old books, like old friends, I swore I would never forget and I had forgotten. The energy wasn't wasted sorting through the past. It helped me let go and get on with life. It helped me recognize the past and give feeling to those unprocessed pieces of the jigsaw puzzle called me. Old decisions and dreams long ago steered me in a direction called now. My constant mantra of "in the future" betrayed so much of my creativity. Now became the time for sorting what gets resurrected and what went into the garbage can. I didn't know how to retire but I was determined to learn.

There was the creativity of planting a new seed and watching a plant rise up out of the soil. There was no guesswork as to what would grow. Then there was creativity in what to plant, what dreams to be realized and some new ones to be created. At that point listening to life became a huge part of my retirement. I watched tomatoes grow in my garden to the point I heard leaves unfurl. My retirement unfurled in the same way. It was cool; cool was an old favorite sixties term. Nature was powerful and I paid attention with reverence more than ever before in my life. I focused on stillness allowing my hand to lie in the dirt for a whole minute without moving it. I felt the moisture and the bugs. The many feeling receptors in the hand were activated. Probably my awareness of receptors increased threefold because I took the time. My new goal was to take time to become more aware, less doing and more listening. Yeah I liked that.

On the flip side I traced things in life that I am most proud of and traced them to thoughts and dreams from the past. My self-reliance didn't happen overnight. Long ago, right or wrong, self-reliance was a seed I sowed. That seed drove me in most of my decisions. I lived the power of that seed thought. In retrospect I would still plant self-reliance but not let it overtake the garden. I was driven and somehow being driven was a seed also. See, so I could throw away or weed out the being driven part and replace it with a listening seed. A seed of listening could not grow in a garden with no space or a space overtaken with being driven.

My prayer became God if I need to know the old dream or belief system let it arise in my consciousness with gentleness and ease. If I don't need to know it let it wash out. In the vacuum created let new relevant dreams take hold in my psyche and may I be led to the next step of seeding, planting and watching the dreams unfold or unfurl like the leaves on the tomato plant. Watching a tomato plant from seedling through bloom to leaves unfurling, to fruit ripening on the vine was a magnificent lesson. I had just planted the retirement seed only there was no picture on any seed packet.

Trust for me was a big challenge. I was more familiar with control. I could trust a tomato plant to grow on its own instead of me controlling it. I fertilized and watered it. Retirement was so personal. If my decision to retire was based in sacredness then my days had to be freeing like the leaves unfurling on the tomato plant. If my decision were based on fear than I would have planted fear and fear would grow. I got it. Plant a tomato get a tomato; plant a sacred seed get sacred; plant fear get fear. Retirement itself may be a seed but more important is what I plant around it; sacredness or fear. I liked this train of thought.

It has been decades since I could decide my daily plans based on my wants rather than requirements. Sure the bill paying and house keeping still took place. But being free in the wind, having the privilege to say yes or no to any request was great. I learned not to be too vocal or happy about my newfound freedom because again nature abhors a vacuum. People heard me being free and thought of it as empty space. People had all types of recommendations to fill my hours with volunteer work etc. I just explained doing nothing is something wonderful especially for a former workaholic. It would have been easier to just make a new job description with a lot of to dos but I choose to take the time to explore and trusted in me to be me.

The main part of my life's definition was my job. It certainly consumed the majority of my free time. My dream now was clearing my psyche of useless thoughts/energy and allowing freedom full reign. If I had possessed a magic wand I would have waved it and made everything negative and unneeded disappear. The reality is that it took time to become truly aware. Even the tomato plant didn't grow from seed to plant overnight. I wanted the joy and awe in the observation, in the journey, and in the fruit.

October 17
Mata Ortiz, Mexico—The Shards of Dreams

My first trip as a retiree was with Elderhostel to Mata Ortiz. Mata Ortiz is a tiny town in Mexico made famous by the internationally know master of pottery. Juan Quazada, His origins were humble and he taught himself how to make pottery. Several years ago I became familiar with his story from lectures at the Heard Museum in Phoenix. When Juan was a youth he would ride his bike through the mountains surrounding Mata Ortiz. Juan did not know about pottery. As he rode on his dilapidated bike, he would stop to pick up bright pieces of broken pottery, which I learned were called shards. The dusty colors caught his attention and he would handle the sharp little pieces of broken clay pots with curiosity. No one in town did pottery and he wasn't quite sure what these little pieces of color were. He only knew he liked touching the clay pieces. His curiosity was peaked and he began questioning the elders of his town. They educated him on what they knew which wasn't much beyond this is pottery.

He saved the shards he found while riding on the mountain paths. His conclusion was if other people did it, he could do it. He knew someone, however long ago, made pots, which had been broken on the mountain. He began piecing the pots together. Many pieces were missing but he got the idea. His imagination delved into color and he returned to the elders questioning their knowledge about coloring clay. There were no good answers so he began his own journey of collecting different colors of clay from the nearby mountains. Thus began his experiment in coloring.

What I loved about Juan's story is his commitment to the town of Mata Ortiz. Once the world discovered he was a master potter he taught the village to mold and fire pottery. In addition to his becoming a success, now the whole town was profiting. Many people who achieve move on and never reach back to their town of birth to train others so they can become successful. It is an inspiring story to me. There were no classes and no one in the whole village knew how to throw or decorate a pot. I was dependent on being taught or at a minimum I required a mentor. Someone always showed up on my path and pointed me in the direction of skill. Juan was dependent on his inner guidance. He asked the questions of elders but he decided what questions to ask. The great majority of people would have picked up the shards and just thrown them away. Juan explored their mystery until he got answers.

Old dreams are the same way. I came across shards in my psyche from long ago and wondered at their meaning or relevance in my life. Some shards were remnants of the collective unconscious and some were from my individual psyche. Around the time of 9/11/01 many people dreamt of airplane accidents in the collective and there was a ton of fear in the aftermath. It became group fear. Individual dreams were more reflective of me or what was specific to me; it might have been my personal fear of a test or getting lost. Whether individual or collective if I wanted to know the meaning I would put the shards together as best I could. I checked with elders. I discovered many things in my research on retirement but something sparked my psyche into desiring experience. The spark for Juan was a simple broken piece of old pottery called a shard.

Juan, because he was listening to his intuition, held onto the shards. Most people would have thrown the pottery shards back on the mountain. Symbolically we all come upon clues to our heart's desires. Some of us have to be hit in the head with a shard before we got it. Many of us didn't take the time to find an elder when we found clues. In my life I have probably ignored tons of shards. I was grateful for the elders who had patience for my questioning. The time for me to look deeper was before me. All I had to do was look and listen to what showed up in my universe.

Presently in Mata Ortiz there are hundreds of new pots made by the residents of this quaint village. Not everyone was drawn to shards but everyone was drawn to something. It would have been easy for Juan to pass by the shards but something deep inside wouldn't let his hand drop the shard. His mind became intrigued and the rest is history. Had he dropped the shard and moved on the world would have missed his art and, I, my lesson about shards. Then again Juan may have picked another path. I know the earth abounds in mystery.

The shards of freedom were in my hands. With full knowledge I planted the freedom seeds in colorful pots; Freedom to listen and to be. My path was not Juan's path or anyone else's path. Each of us is here for different reasons. Had I ridden my bike on the mountains of Mata Ortiz I would have zipped past the shards and that would have been perfect for me. Pottery is not my calling.

I granted myself permission to review all my old dreams and to gather up any missed symbolic shards. I may have missed some signs along the way but it is never too late to begin. The Mata Ortiz shards taught me freedom to resurrect old dreams and to sharpen my awareness of shards on my path.

November 1
Kitchen—Monkey See Monkey Do

Somewhere, somehow, I allowed a thought of kitchen remodeling to enter my mind. Those thoughts entered from the side through a tiny peephole and grew into big expensive payments. So be it. I explored my neighbor's newly remodeled kitchen and thought wouldn't it be nice to actually move through my kitchen without bruising my legs. In the original design of my house there were two cabinets that jutted out from the kitchen wall blocking the entryway into the dining room. This was actually presented to me as a feature of the house. That began the rationalization process for remodeling. Within six months of retiring I gutted my kitchen. Instead of a fancy trip to Europe I remodeled my kitchen. It was my retirement trip. What a deal. My human mind was so quick to rationalize. So I cleaned out cabinets and selected colors.

I've never been much of a cook so it was a whole new world. My pantry was full of papers and non-food related items. Through the years my pantry was a filing cabinet of non-food items, mostly gifts and paperwork. Prior to becoming a file cabinet my pantry was the emptiest cabinet in the house. I even unearthed a long forgotten box of Shakespeare books that I had purchased in Indiana at a library sale.

Negotiating with kitchen contractors was another challenge. It reminded me of bargaining with kids except kids are more honest. Once I had a contract in place workers showed up at my house. While they worked in the kitchen I was busy in the alley with my tomato garden. The alleys between the houses in central Phoenix were not officially used for city business so homeowners utilized the area. Permanent structures were not allowed. Shortly after I fertilized, planted seeds and watered little shoots burst through the dirt. All plants are a miracle to me and especially anything that can grow in my alley.

During the kitchen transformation I watched tomatoes grow and pulled weeds. It was an art to relax. To literally sit and do nothing took practice. I envisioned so many other things in my house that needed attention and cleaning. I decided my heart needed the silence, the peace and quiet to just be with the alley garden. Fourteen plants became my focus and I expected them to produce hundreds of tomatoes. My coffee maker got moved to the carport and was conveniently filled and plugged in all morning. Neighbors walking their dogs and curious neighbors stopped for a cup of brew and heard the latest about my kitchen and neighborhood news. Dogs got a fresh drink of water. The tomato garden received a lot of comment and positive thoughts. At first it floored me that I sat doing nothing and it drew so much attention from neighbors. I explained watching tomatoes grow was something. They were used to me busy with lists of things to do. It was my norm. My lists typically continued into the next day and the next day. It was foreign to just sit and be me. It became fun and empowered me to realize freedom. Choosing to be rather than do all the time sounded simple. It was complex.

Most articles about preparing for retirement suggested that a new retiree skip or postpone remodeling in the first year of retirement. Remodeling could be stressful. The task became grounding because I chose to stay home as the work transpired. The noise of workers in my house forced me, and my coffee pot, outside. I went with the flow. Had the kitchen people not been in my house I would have found something else to do. Nothing could have been better for me than sitting and watching tomatoes grow. It slowed me down enough to let me be aware of me. Choosing to upgrade my kitchen was the fulfillment of an old dream. Only it led to something far more important than my kitchen. It led me to awareness of seeds growing into plants and fruiting. The seeds of my thoughts and my freedom worked the same way.

New kitchen meant new appliances and pans. My dilemma was either selecting all new appliances or keeping an older theme to match my 1965 stove. I choose modern and even selected a double door refrigerator with an icemaker. The rationale I used to purchase new was retirement is a one shot deal. Celebrate it once and in high fashion. Some people bought motor homes and started traveling. Some, like me, transformed kitchens. Maybe it was a nesting thing because I had no plan or desire to travel.

Monkey see, monkey do, and monkey speak. I became a consultant to friends on kitchen remodeling. It was short-lived but a worthy experience nonetheless. The shard that led to my kitchen became an expression of freedom. In my gutted kitchen I stood and began imagining what it would look like completed. It was cool. Pen in hand I wrote peace, harmony, love, and wisdom on the bare walls. The words got painted over. It was wonderful knowing these words surrounded and enfolded my kitchen. Invisible now but I knew the words were there under the paint. I cooked with wisdom and peace. A dear friend gave me handmade tiles that read peace, love, trust, and hope. I hung them over the kitchen sink. Every time I wash my hands or dishes I read them. Words manifest. I am so grateful for the symbolic shard or dream that lead to a new kitchen in my life.

December 10
Grand Canyon Hiking—Initiating the Journey of the Healing Mountain

When a person signs up for Elderhostel she receives all kinds of literature on Elderhostel trips all over the world. It was wonderful to think of all the possibilities. Before I left for Mata Ortiz I signed up for the Grand Canyon hike. I thought it would be a good spiritual retreat to celebrate my first year of retirement. It required I get into good hiking shape. The thin people in the promotional hiking photo made me realize the strenuousness of getting into shape. Each person in the photo held sticks or poles. These were trekking poles. I was intimidated by my lack of knowledge. Years ago I hiked the Bright Angel and Kaibob trails at the south rim of the Grand Canyon. In my fifties and fifty pounds heavier it was going to be a challenge.

Once I returned from Mata Ortiz I looked for a mountain in Phoenix that was climbable for a novice. Thunderbird Mountain became the spot. A friend introduced me to the mountain and we hiked. It took three hours with many, many stops. I was exhausted and felt healthy mentally and physically. Climbing Thunderbird became a ritual. What a pleasure it was to observe I hiked while others worked. It hit home, I was able to do what I wanted to do. Hiking trails on the mountain were basically empty and I became a regular. There were about twelve of us. The mountain changed with the weather. It became vibrant with wildflowers and mystical during thunderstorms. It was amazing to watch my physical body change with the frequency of climbs. I dropped twenty-five pounds and my mind was freer than it had been in years.

Freedom was a mystery. To practice freedom moment-by-moment was hard for me because I had so many regrets about the past and anxiety about the future that cropped up. I kicked these unproductive thoughts out of my mind and listened to the present moment with an open heart. When one is loosed of the past and the future, one can listen with an open heart. Too many times I have missed what was happening in the present moment because of being caught up in the past or the future. My mind was cleared of tasks and to do lists while I hiked because I deemed it so. This freed me to sense the mountain through the rocks, the animals, and the flowers. It inspired me to watch the water run down the mountain during a rainstorm. It wasn't so exciting to hear a rattlesnake slither on the trail but I took the time to feel and look with all my senses. My heart felt the joy welling up inside me as I held a rock or watched an insect. It amazed me what learning can take place in the silence.

People talked on the trail and many an interesting conversation occurred on the mountaintop. It was a sacred space of truth. In the distance a mountain that looked like an Indian's face stared up at the sky with a tear falling down its cheek. I saw horses, burros, snakes, bunnies, and even a swarm of bees. Thunderbird Mountain was my healing mountain.

It was time for the Grand Canyon trip. Being from Arizona I second-guessed myself as to why I chose this trip rather than some foreign exotic place. The canyon was beyond words. I never saw the same thing twice even though my eyes looked twice at the same spot. The magnitude of the canyon was incomprehensible and a picture did not do it justice. It was like trying to catch life in a photo. The effect could be caught but the actual experience would be limited in a snapshot.

The hiking was great and the weather cool. One day when the Grand Canyon group hiked down the Kaibob trail the sun was relentless and hotter than normal for December. Arizona sun is hot everyday period. My top layer of a coat and a second layer of a sweatshirt got stuffed in my backpack within a half hour. My bottom layer was a black turtleneck and black hiking pants. The hotter I got the redder my face became until it felt like I was going to pass out. I asked for and, fortunately, the trail guide had scissors. I cut the collar off my turtleneck, made it sleeveless and cut away the midriff section just below my bra. My belly stood out. My outfit resembled a Goodwill reject. I looked like something the cat dragged in but it was okay with me. I was happy and much cooler.

December 17
The Single Matrix

A single never married heterosexual woman is a rare species. I generally don't fit into social equations easily. I believe there is a balance between work, risk, and trust that I just didn't get. I learned to trust the integrity of my soul because it was my path. I learned in a Steven Levine workshop a phrase; "the healing we took birth for" and it resonated with me. That phrase interpreted to me that each of us came for a reason. Some of us completed it in one year of life and others it may take one hundred years. Time doesn't matter in eternity. The healing could be in relationship, in creation like the Mata Ortiz pottery or in a healing of the heart. It might relate to past lives or events in this life. All the accumulation of things wasn't as important as the "healing we took birth for." I honor the phrase because it reminded me that I don't have to judge or understand other people's choices. Each person's path was different. The concept of free will fascinated me. Instead of giving free will to all I wanted people to do what I wanted them to do rather than allow them free will. I didn't know anyone else's purpose. I didn't even know mine but I was headed in the direction of learning.

The part of my brain that rationalized anything popped up to claim responsibility for my life choices. I chose it, it didn't choose me. There were many opportunities to marry but for whatever reason I made other choices. The single matrix made a difference. Bargains were galore for couples. Friends of mine who roam the country in motor homes as couples receive many discounts. Not so for my single friends, they got to pay supplements. Thank God driving around the country never appealed to me. I got lost in a paper bag and I had no desire to drive anything longer than my jeep. Shared costs with another single could have been beneficial but I snored and preferred my own space. There were no discounts for snorers. It was cheaper and more convenient to be a couple. Nothing major but financially being single made a difference.

My pondering was pointing me to wanting this illusive, to me, intimate relationship. In my past I had the Cinderella dreams of happily ever after but the reality in my life was workaholic. For an old feminist work was a definer. I believed intimacy and freedom were mutually exclusive which is false. I like to believe intimacy was welcomed in my life.

There are certain advantages in being single. I didn't need approval. I woke up and went to sleep when I wanted. My journey in learning responsibility was expedited by being single. There was no one else to blame. Some people in intimate relationships comment they can't be free and feel trapped because of responsibilities to the kids/grandkids. The same people later say "I wouldn't be able to get by without the support of my kids/grandkids, they keep me going." So much of life's purpose is reproducing and loving the children. Some believe that procreating is their only purpose. Many people, like me, without children have other purposes. Many people with children have purposes in addition to their children. Being good parents was just their major purpose. I pondered that shard of information. I trusted the intelligence of the universe. Even if no one knew the specifics, there was purpose to every life and every breath.

My choices had been serial monogamy with long in betweens of abstinence. Retirement put a whole new focus on things. I was going to have time for a lot more activity. The time and space of deep conversation and soul searching was another spark of desire. An intimate other would be fun. Intimacy showed up in many ways in my life. In retrospect I was afraid of someone actually seeing the real me. I was so grateful for friendships. I supposed this decision to not marry had been the shard for the depth of my spiritual journey. I knew it wasn't the only way but it became my way.

I love these shards. It is like a tiny piece of a large puzzle fell at my feet. I pick the piece up and imagine what the whole picture looked like with all the pieces together. If the shard resonated with my soul then it became a mission to piece it together. Otherwise I let it go. A shard was a piece of Humpty Dumpty in the dirt. With no other pieces I knew it was part of something larger. I tried putting Humpty together again with just one piece and no picture. I felt successful because I knew the single piece was important to me and led to something. This shard of intimacy felt uncomfortable because it was foreign. I had no idea what the final picture would look like. The exploration of the puzzle pieces called intimacy became comfortable because I liked adventure. It felt right to keep the shard even though it was one tiny piece. To throw it away or ignore it wasn't a choice.

January 8
Beginning Watercolor Class

Somewhere in my memory bank were remembrances of art classes in grade school taught by nuns. I colored pictures of saints or baby Jesus. I had no memory of art classes in high school. So in my fifties I took an art class at a community college and felt insecure to say the least. It was a weekday morning class for the privileged non-working of which I was a part. I was thrilled to be in it and now I wanted to see what I could do. A friend and I took the class together. Doing art is a single alone journey. It is within my individual psyche where decisions are made and implemented. These decisions transformed a blank sheet of paper into something. Out of the nothingness creativity was born. Life is like that. Ideas come out of the darkness or silence. I was born with <u>tabla rosa,</u> a blank slate, and then with my first breath of life it all began. Even if one believes in reincarnation, there is a blank slate at birth. Yeah and one could argue boundaries between this life and past lives. It challenged my brain to think of the possibilities. I liked the cleanliness of a blank slate and knew I made the decisions as to what got painted and how I reacted to what I painted.

Back to art class, the first day I brought to class all the required materials to a tune of two hundred dollars. The class tuition itself was only seventy-eight dollars. There were about a dozen or so other students and several arrived with paintings in hand that I categorized as Picassos. As a retiree I learned not to judge myself and that I was fine wherever I was and whatever I was doing. It was like belonging to a sorority of self-acceptance knowing I earned a place in the sisterhood of being satisfied right where I was. There was no boss or fellow employees. The response from others when I said I was retired was generally "you are so lucky." I knew and tried not to gloat. Years ago I shied away from putting myself in an art class because I feared failure. My courage to explore new things increased dramatically because I was less likely to care about other people's judgment of me. I knew it was all okay and being a beginner at anything is part of exploring. It was all okay. As long as I was learning I didn't care how others judged or didn't judge me.

So my first day in class we did water scenes which was fun. It was amazing how a long wide, curvy brushstroke of blue water-color on paper actually resembled water flowing in a stream. Next we moved to flowers, poppies to be exact. I was much better painting the abstract. When it had to actually look like something I was challenged. My flowers were botanically incorrect; there were too many strokes inside the center of the flower. It looked like a hundred sticks blooming inside a flower. Next we did trees and I have an affinity for trees. Trees are more forgiving. Trees aren't perfect. Their branches bend and are irregular in shape. Their color is inconsistent and the color varied by season. Small animals and insects lived in trees so a mishap with my paintbrush became a bug. Nothing was uniform about a tree. Mistakes were less likely to be noticed by my untrained eye. Using the word mistake wasn't accurate. My paintbrush revealed what could exist on a blank piece of paper with just a little paint and my hand set free. I thought my conscious mind was directing everything. In reality my unconscious was being heard. If my painting was choppy then I knew I was too controlling. When my brush just glided the results were prettier and more recognizable. When my mind just flowed it was powerful.

My favorite part of the class utilized spattered India ink. It was an exercise in letting loose reminiscent of kindergarten art with freedom for finger-paint fun. My watercolor teacher had us cover the floor with old newspapers to catch the mess. Then we watched as the teacher dipped a razor blade into a cat food can filled with India ink. She appeared reckless as she flung the ink from the blade onto a large sheet of white paper. Her quick wrist action was followed by a quick swish or swipe of the blade on the paper. After it dried we gathered around the ink spattering and identified what we saw in the design. Some saw flowers, some water, but the winner for the day was the student who saw sail boats in the ink pattern. The teacher picked up her watercolors with brush and painted transforming the splotches into a sailing scene. Her skilled hands painted around the ink utilizing every inch of the ink into a sailboat scene. It amazed me and reminded me what one found when one looked for something, for anything. Now it was the students' turn and we followed the teacher's example and dipped our razors into the India ink and new splotches were born.

It was fun pouring India ink into a cat food can and dipping the razor blade into it. Then it was my turn. I overdid the splotching on my first try. My white sheet was black with ink. There wasn't any space in between splotches.

My second attempt was better with considerable more white space. I walked around and looked from all four directions but I had no idea what my design was. My pep talk to myself was I am retired and I could try anything. This time when I turned the paper I saw a woman's face in what was a wisp of a tree. Her face, half hidden, emerged from what was an outline of a tree. With browns and greens I begun the journey of painting the white spaces and uncovered her hidden in the splotches. Life happened in the white and ink space. In the end the teacher said my painting was spiritual. She could have meant many things but I loved my painting. It is framed and hangs over my fireplace. People make comments like "what is this" or "the woman in the tree needs a dentist." I believe she winks through it all. The painting was baptized "The Tree Nymph." What began as shards of India ink splotches morphed into a tree nymph. With no judgment or negativity it is what it is. Years ago it would have been hidden because it wasn't deemed perfect. Retirement was sacred. As one friend put it I had lost my need for perfection.

January 15
Motor Home a New Language

Just about every retired person hears motor home language. It has a vocabulary all its own. I wondered about the location of an interpretive dictionary. My friends had a motor home; in fact, they just bought a second camping trailer for shorter trips. With both motor home and camping trailer in their yard they questioned if both covered their needs. The smaller camping trailer couldn't accommodate four days of food. It was good for two days. The motor home was optimal for trips longer than a week. It was retirement language. My mind looked for the closest restaurant not the amount of food packed. As my fiends traveled they learned many card games that they taught me. Hand/Foot and Mexican Train Ride are a couple of examples. When I pulled in their driveway I was greeted by the smaller camping trailer with the porch awning opened up ready for camp. I got the sense of being out in the open spaces of nature. It had to be freeing to just pack up and go without the need to plan hotels and restaurants. It was down to earth and homey just to get behind that wheel and go. My ideal was one of those homes with a chauffer freed of duty upon arrival at my destination. It was like my abandoned desire for a self-cleaning house. As my friend put it, I was recognizing that preference was not necessarily limitation. Everything exists and was possible.

February 10
Retirement Homes—My Age

Fleeting thoughts about retirement homes crossed my mind and were always met with not for me but for someone else. Another neighbor invited me to attend a meeting with him at a local retirement community. A new addition to the existing facility was the subject. My neighbor just passed the ninety-year-old mark. He had become familiar with the facility because his father, back in the eighties, lived there. The presentation amazed me. All levels of assistance with matching price tags were available. The crux would be to know when to move and how to pay. I didn't think I ever heard of anyone who moved too soon. Many paid too much. I guessed I would be in denial with my head stuck in the sand when my time came. It had to be the hardest decision to accept inability to live independently. It left me speechless.

My neighbor and I arrived at the senior facility for the sales presentation. To his joy they updated on the four on site restaurants. Personal choice was a thing of the sixties; it was front and center for us baby boomers. Generations who came of age during the depression or world wars didn't have as much an opportunity to know personal choices. Freedom in personal choices is easier in times of affluence. What I did with my new found freedom was the first and foremost question people asked me. It seemed my age was in a catch area and brought up people's old belief systems about retirement. Many associated retirement with illness and loss of will. I was happy to be free and healthy. Health challenges decreased one's ability to enjoy retirement. Financial health was also a factor. Travel was an option. Freedom to be me was more important than any trip. Trips were a nice addition but not the main dish

Gardens are a new and beautiful addition to any home and they seemed to be a big thing in the renovation phase of this senior facility. It was stated several times during the ninety-minute presentation. I could envision myself focused on gardening wherever I lived.

All my old belief systems about retirement and nursing homes came to the surface. I had visions of bedsores and no food. I needed to update my old ways of thinking because old unhealthy belief systems caused negativity and depression. I decided to let amazement at what I didn't know guide me. After the marketing pitch we meandered through the grounds. We came upon two sweet talkative little ladies with new coiffures done on site in the local beauty parlor. They directed us to the formal dining room with its large windows that overlooked the flower garden. This was a nice place to wind down when life was coming to a close. My denial reared its head. I surmised that I learned more about my denials. I negated any exploration of me living here in the near future. Later maybe, but certainly not now.

March 8
Master Gardener Class

An old friend suggested I take a master gardener class. He had just completed the class and talked about how much fun it had been and how many wonderful people he had met. People like us who were newly retired. Nature was a great teacher. How a tree could grow from a tiny seed was inspiring. Knowing that the thoughts planted in my psyche did the same thing, revealed much. I had always heard the tree was in the seed before the tree was in the ground. One couldn't help but wonder at what had been planted to grow an oak tree. It was just like in the garden. Look at what grew to know what was planted. It was why I keep the thought of sacred and retirement always connected. It kept me accountable.

I learned most people over water and over prune their trees. I believed I overdid watering because I couldn't stand the thought of deprivation. The thought of trees suffering without water had to reflect my past times of doing without. It was probably my poor attempt at rescuing a tree. Over watering might have drowned a tree. Some insects were good for the garden and some were not. Fertilizing and mulch played an important part in the garden. In the desert we had sun and more sun. One could use desert-adapted plants or import trees and shrubs from back east. Trees from back east wasted a lot of water. It sounded like sabotage to bring plants from back east but many people did it. Some people moved to the desert and then tried to change the desert rather than become adapted. In retirement some became so busy with "doing" they didn't and couldn't adapt to the idea or lifestyle of retirement. If I wanted a back east lifestyle then I needed to move back east. If I wanted a working lifestyle then I needed to go to work. Volunteer work and doing what I love isn't work it is pure joy.

The earth gave via the garden. I thought I had so much to do with the gardening process because I prepared soil, selected the seeds, and planted them. It was pure earth, unseen to the naked eye, which evolved the seed into a pepper or a tomato. I imagined what I might be like if I planted myself into the earth as a "joy of retirement" seed. I would grow into a joyous happy retiree. The quantum field accepted my request and I allowed it to come forth. In the quantum field the universe responded. Branches with leaves of joy sprouted from my spine like a tree sapling sprouting branches. My journey found what joy looked and felt like. It felt like when I painted the ink splotches, like I had solved a mystery about my life. I knew how to be me. Boiled down it appeared I found happiness in the present moment in wherever I was and in whatever I did. My happiness did not depend on anything outside myself. The route of retirement wasn't the only route for me to learn but it was my personal way to discover my passions.

March 12
Freedom to be Wrong—Thundering into the Sunrise

Sometimes I was more interested in being right than anything else. And sometimes I just hung on and wanted a clean stead before I made a clear-cut decision. There were many times I allowed myself to feel responsible for other people's feelings and reactions. I became this giant screen for their projections. I could have asked them to own and rewind their projections off me and to project them somewhere else if they couldn't own them but I didn't. My goal became being so free to state what was on my mind. Being authentic, right or wrong, was important to me. I was obsessed over erroneous quality. I obsessed about leaving a clean stead. A friend called it ego and said I wanted to be liked by everyone. It was the wrong definition of nice. To put it into perspective several months ago I decided I had been part of a social group for too long. My decision was long overdue. I hadn't noticed that I had grown in another direction. Belonging to the group was comfortable because it was routine and no thinking was necessary. I decided to discontinue membership. This upset several people and I allowed their upset to affect my decision to leave. It felt as if I was uprooting my seed from deep within the earth. You know when you have planted something new and instead of waiting for it to grow you dig it up and then get upset because it did not bloom. That was me. I rationalized to myself that I was of too great assistance to be leaving and that definitely was my big ego. It was all okay and I granted myself permission to be wrong. That was freedom. In the past my being wrong would have brought up guilt and lots of it. The mystery of freedom wasn't so easy.

Freedom is an awesome thing. It meant being free to speak even if wrong about what I had to say. This group had become a safe oasis for me and it was time to move on. It had been a blessing and a safe place to hide. I needed to grow and follow my seed of joy. Sometimes it was best to just sit still during a group meeting and not say a word. It was like being in meditation. Some people called it being smart. Other times it was appropriate to be active in the meeting and to respond or react. There was so much judgment under the guise of morals, which in my mind was the anti-Christ. Silence was perceived as a very wise thing and was actually quite easy. If someone asked for spirit within the meeting then silence was wise. Silence wasn't possible if I was thick in discussion. It was hard to actively participate and be silent at the same time. I told my friend that this time instead of a written letter of resignation to the group I was going to fade wordless into the sunset. Her response was that I needed to ride out in style not fade away. Riding out in control of the horse named emotion, she said, was more my style than silence. My freedom to be wrong led me to change fading into the sunset to thundering into the sunrise with words. A definite new belief system began for me. Being retired gave me the opportunity to contemplate these things. Consistency in the brain was a good thing. Sunrise in the morning announced the beginning of the day. Thundering was the sound of horses coming up over a hill entering a new terrain. Unafraid and free the state of the stead became irrelevant. All these things were available in the universe whether or not I was retired. It was just easier since I was retired. Retirement translated to more choices. Somewhere I read that the Dali Lama observed that a cat whenever the opportunity presents itself would slide out a cracked window. That is the power of freedom. I left and the group was better than ever. And I was happier. Staying to please others or what I perceived to be pleasing others would have been a big mistake. It wouldn't have been good for the group or me.

March 15
Dreams

The dream world has always fascinated me. There were dream interpreters in the bible and many dream interpreters in this day and age. The most powerful dream interpreter in my opinion is the dreamer. In order to remember my dreams I had to train my mind. Prior to sleep I told myself three things, I wanted to wake up after a dream, remember the dream, and have the energy to record it either on my tape recorder or with pen/pad. It didn't work to interpret the dream while dreaming or when first awake. If I didn't program myself to have the energy to keep awake while recording the dream my conscious mind told me my dream wasn't important and I would quickly return to sleep. Returning to sleep was an easier option. The dream was forgotten. There is much information in my dreams, which is why I began recording them years ago. Tracking dream symbols helped me interpret the meaning of my dreams. My subconscious mind did not know language, only symbols. Dreams arose from my subconscious. Some dreams symbols had universal meaning and some were specific to me as the dreamer.

In deciding on when to retire I recorded every remembered dream. One night I had a lengthy dream full of clean towels. Both of my parents (now deceased) were in the dream. My father said nothing but nodded with a knowing smile. The dream involved burning buildings. My mother gave me a dog on a leash. Later she threw me a baby from a burning building as I prepared to escape the fire. I caught the baby. My mother unafraid stayed behind and I left with the baby. My father was just outside the gate of the city. It was a very peaceful departure in spite of the chaos occurring within the fiery city. It was like the Phoenix bird silently rising from the ashes. The next morning after thought and coffee my decision to retire was clear. I began preparing.

Dreams are powerful. Not every dream is major. Many were just processing minor things that had occurred during my day. Turning television off and drifting to sleep with a question on my mind lead me to a responsive dream. Someone, whose name I can't remember, suggested that the question of the dreamer was like a large bucket lowered into a well (the subconscious mind) and the bucket filled with the answer. Upon awakening the dream bucket was raised up for viewing at the surface of the conscious mind. In an instant the dream was remembered but as consciousness awakened the bucket with its dream content returned and re-entered the well mixing once again into the subconscious. The dream then would likely never be remembered. The window of opportunity to remember the dream is short. Once I returned to consciousness the dream was gone. Dreaming about thundering horses would be fun. The dream state has no filters.

Entry April 1
The Muumuu Club

When I was growing up I thought wearing muumuus was a right of passage for women becoming old. My mother and every one else's mother wore them. Watching someone wearing a muumuu was like watching someone wear a tent in bright colors jiggle down the street. They are great cover-ups. So when some female friends and I found ourselves as new retirees meeting for lunch and movies we founded the muumuu club. We were different than our moms and retirement was certainly different in the 2000s than it was in the 1970s. Our goal as muumuus was eat lunch and see a movie. It was a very mature gathering for newly retired females. And we vowed never to own a muumuu because if we wore a muumuu we would be old like we thought our mothers were back then. We discussed a possible muumuu handshake and theme song but never made a decision.

One can learn a lot by laughing together. We discussed and laughed at our past mistakes. The things we thought were so important dimmed when we saw them with a new perception. It was laughable what we told ourselves. It was great to have a place to be safe from judgment as we discussed personal issues.

My muumuu club gave me the freedom to be silly. I wondered sometimes if these types of clubs were just for a moment and not worthy of the title club. As a child being a member of a club held a mystique. I thought someone who belonged to a club was special and hand picked. The assumption I made was that not everyone could get into that club. It's another old belief system that needed to be released into the nothingness. This process cleared the way for a new belief system to spring up. For right now I was privileged and honored to be a member of the muumuu club. There was no shard along the way just pure laughter.

Entry April 9
Travel

Retirement and travel are not synonymous even though they popped up in many conversations as a natural link. Most retirees talked about a possible retirement trip. My money for a trip was used for remodeling my kitchen.

When I was working and went on vacation the first two or three days were spent resting and unwinding. About the fourth day I would start thinking about work and what was waiting for me when I returned to the office. Many times I remembered flying back to Phoenix feeling dread in my gut about vacation being over. I took a short trip not long after I retired and when I flew back to Phoenix it was the first time I returned as a retiree. Indescribable joy welled up in me because I knew I did not have to return to work. Work as I knew it was over. I could compare that feeling to hearing my name read as a winner of a million dollar jackpot. So much of my past was routine hours, routine church, routine cards etc. Now nothing was routine. There was this ease about scheduling myself. If I felt I was overscheduled I breathed into "wow I am free to do or not do." That freedom was worth a great deal to me. Sometimes I questioned if my pension matched my financial needs. I reminded myself that my expenditures were not flamboyant. The fear was not valid. It was an old fear of not having enough.

More doors of potential opened in my psyche upon retiring. In the past the doors were sealed shut with a red sticker that read, "later when you retire." Travel was possible twelve months out of the year. I was not pinned down to a specific two-week period. An option of three months in Ireland was possible. My brain flashed I don't want to be out of the country three months. Going to Ireland for three months was a seed planted long ago but it wasn't still a desire. Desires change through the years and living an old desire can be a deterrent to enjoying the present. Those old beliefs can be released, making space for new dreams. I would gladly trade in the old prom dress dream from years ago for a summer cabin. A new dream for me would be having a summer cabin in northern Arizona. Consciousness expanded with new ideas and concepts. The psyche always expanded and filled large empty spaces. Maybe that was why churches are so big especially in Europe. Spirit filled those spaces and impacted our hearts and minds with open spaces.

I concluded that freedom needed a place to grow and expand. Traveling was certainly an option because it opened the horizon to new things. Changes would lead to expansion. Traveling was a good way, but not the only way.

Entry April 21
Sex—Take it or Leave it

I examined my previous perceptions of young females dressing for school. Some had no inhibition. Aside from the fact I attended catholic schools I wouldn't have been caught dead with my bra strap showing or wearing white clothes after Labor Day. Without judgment I was awestruck by these young people wearing what would have been called slutty in my day. Sadly for many youth today it is a call for attention that draws inappropriate attention. Look at the Internet scenarios of forty-year-old men who met and abused underage teenage boys and girls.

There are examples of teachers engaged in sexual violations with young students. It was not even unusual to hear of female teachers violating underage male students. A recent example was the female teacher who was impregnated by her student. She was sentenced to jail, was released, and broke a court order that prohibited her from seeing him. She was now married to this young man who had become an adult and they now have two children. Freedom could be wisely and unwisely used. Sex with a minor is illegal. Marrying a legal adult after having had illegal sex with him as a minor was not illegal. It could or could not be love. It was none of my business and obviously not the court's business. They both had freedom to choose as adults.

I have heard lots of great sexy stories in retirement communities. The people there, like me, are retired not dead. The word tired is in retired. All one had to do was watch television and observe all the ads for sex enhancing drugs. The target market for these drugs is older adults. They aren't recommended for young people who supposedly didn't need them but used them anyway for kicks. We are a country of sexual prowess. I don't know where I missed the boat but I did. I immersed myself in the free love society back in the sixties but didn't participate in the activities. I loved the freethinking but I was heavily enmeshed in the Catholic traditions of fear and guilt. In the late sixties and early seventies I lived in Berkeley and Boston. It was an inspirational time of creativity and I am glad I chose it.

I do regret not experimenting more with sex. I feel like the brother to the Prodigal Son. I did what was supposed to be done and remained abstinent. In the Prodigal story the brother felt cheated when the prodigal returned and received the same reward as he who towed the line of supposed righteousness. My view of sex was skewed. I, like the brother in the prodigal story, followed the right path, and felt repressed. I missed the exploration. I will never know if I am better or worse for that decision. My sexual immaturity and inexperience may have made me more open to betrayal.

Sex in the traveling motor home population was ripe for a best selling novel or a television series like "Peyton Place on wheels." Some of us baby boomers burnt bras, fought for equal rights, participated in free love, experimented with birth control and joined the mile high club. I wonder what the future years hold for seniors in the sexual arena. My generation birthed a creative burst of energy in the sixties. Sex wouldn't be business as usual. They called it Grey Power or the AARP generation. Instead of "Sex in the City" it could be "Sex for Seniors." For most it wasn't sex for sex. Sex, I believed as I aged, was more about healthy connection and non-sexual intimacy then it was about the actual sex. Many men have had prostrate surgery and are no longer engaged in normal sexual activity but they remained intimate. There are other ways to have sex and this senior generation forged another path. Women in the past have had hysterectomies and their sexual reproductive organs have been removed. Many a time it was a horror story of just yanking out organs while they were opened for surgery anyway. They wouldn't be bearing more children so their organs were yanked. The baby boomer generation showed the value of something greater than sex and that was real love. We have gone full gamut in the realm of sex. This is true for all of us wherever we are on the spectrum of sexuality be that gay, lesbian, straight, trans, bi or whatever else exists.

A bit off the story but in 1979 during a long weekend we took a day trip to Cherry Grove on Fire Island in New York. It was a wild place and a favorite party spot for the gay population. Heterosexuals were also drawn because the bands blared and everything represented freedom, beauty, and wildness. It was way over the top on the scale of wild. In the late 1990s I read an article in the New York Times that Cherry Grove had become a safe haven for the people, the gay people, who suffered from AIDS. What a transformation! This gay population taught me a lot by example. The place of wildness had become sacred. I wondered if that was true for everything. Compassion would have the last word. May my heart be free to transform. I would have loved to participate in that change at Cherry Grove. It brought back a memory of me returning to graduate school in Manhattan after my wild brief 1979 weekend on Fire Island. On the bus ride to the subway station I sat behind two young men sharing a very intimate kiss; they gazed longingly in each other's eyes and seemed to know their kiss couldn't continue once they returned to New York. They literally pulled apart from each other. It was sad but powerful in its honesty of having to hide. May compassion have the last word. Before retirement I would have wanted to focus on time and efficiency. Now I flowed. I was free to flow. The shards were everywhere.

Entry April 26
Church Redefined

I used to think that when buildings read, "Church" that was church; self-contained within the walls. Some claim church is a place to gather. Others said God is everywhere and not limited to any religion or geographic location. The location was irrelevant. I was reminded of that yesterday. I finished my hike. Some people at the end of the trail passed out bottled water as part of their community church project. The free ice-cold bottle of water in my hot sweaty hands at the end of a four-mile hike on a hot afternoon was a gift. The bottle read "Horizons Community Church" and quoted John 4:13-14 "Everyone who drinks of this water shall thirst again; but whoever drinks of the water I shall give him shall never thirst, but the water I shall give him shall become in him a well of water springing up to eternal life." The cold water itself was refreshing. It wasn't the container or even the water in the bottle that inspired me. It was the message that got my attention. Nourishment came in many forms. The gay population on Fire Island did just what the message stated. They nourished the spirit in addition to the body. I held the bottle and knew the people on Fire Island understood this message and they taught me. The message resonated in my mind long after the water quenched my thirst.

Some people think church is a building with a set of rules. A lot of people include praying silently or swinging a golf club in their definition of church. Some churches prayed with enthusiasm and love. In Religious Science the founder, Ernest Holmes, said, "Change your thinking change your life." Many of my spiritual teachers taught me living life was an inside job. When a new thought was planted and accepted in my psyche things changed. Too often my thoughts were negative and negative results occurred. Observing my thoughts was especially challenging to me. My mind wandered and all sorts of ideas and judgments came up. Pleasing people isn't a noble goal. Being kind and loving in response to people's opinions of me was noble.

Sometimes being kind and loving required confrontation. Many years ago I read in the book titled "The Road Less Traveled" something to the effect that not confronting what needed to be confronted was abuse. Things like manipulation are so easy to hide under the cloak of caring. Confronting the unknown or hidden agendas is challenging. Look at predators of children who started out as helpful to the child. In reality the predator was manipulating the innocence of the child. There are a few examples of church members who manipulated the innocence of members. Look at suicide bombers and priests who abused. They may be in the minority but they got the publicity. There are many wonderful Muslims I've met and it is painful to see what the few misguided souls under the guise of being Muslim accomplished. In my own life there were times I allowed myself to be led down the wrong path. It was frustrating. I had an old belief system that said vulnerability decreased with age and that wasn't true. Seniors get bilked out of thousands of dollars because they trust the wrong companies and people. We all know lots of examples. The point was that churches are not immune from being manipulative and dishonest. At one time I thought all churches were honest and moved in integrity. The majority of churches may be on the up and up but certainly it is not a hard fast rule. Church to me is more how I lived and included being on the golf course. Age didn't exempt me from thievery. Being older makes me a possible target. I thought I was wiser. I don't want to get lazy in my thinking. With the freedom of retirement I guarded against being lax by not thinking.

Entry May 1
Politics

There is no place, other than the coffin, where politics did not rear its head. Just like money and anything else, politics are used for good or bad. The same mind power that Adolph Hitler utilized to hurt a race is the same power I utilized for positive thinking. Young children don't bother too much with politics, they just grab what they want and there is no hiding. As one ages we became politically astute and then we revert, I guess, to a second childhood. It all works out because in the end the spirit is all that matters. I doubt that politics play a role in spirit. I liked to watch Meet the Press and was amazed at Tim Russert. He was a smart guy and handled a political round table like no body's business. I worried when a guest spoke about Washington D.C. needing to learn what the rest of the country knew. People speak from our capitol and don't have a pulse on the country. It is a sad state of affairs when the capitol doesn't know what is happening. We elected people to know. AARP certainly knew how to gather and politicize seniors. They began gathering us as we turned fifty. That was very smart.

We use politics in our families, in our churches, and in our jobs. It is everywhere. It could be consumer friendly if one knew what was wanted and how to get it. Recently I disappointed someone who put me up on a pedestal. Intellectually I knew the placement wasn't fair but I honored and respected the person. Emotional people are susceptible to being manipulated. If someone knows you don't like to get upset all they have to do is threaten you with upset and you would go along. Show a child starving in a foreign country and we're all moved. It is a compliment to humanity that we care. Yet someone with ill intentions could manipulate that situation into money for personal gain at the real expense of the starving children. It is wise not to be lax in my judgment in retirement. My point is to think and not be ruled by emotions. Politics and emotions are a deadly combination. When emotion takes over, logic goes out the window and it is the end of discussion.

I think future senior centers can be more consumer friendly to a hip older generation. It would be natural to gather the energies of seniors in places where they went for fun. In New York City neighborhoods are politically powerful units and in Phoenix that became a reality. The City Council in Phoenix was composed of eight citywide representatives elected at large in a general election. Now the city is divided into eight geographic locations and each area has elected its own representative. There is a specific person for an area rather than all the council people serving the city at large. For the life of me I have never figured out why some one would want to run for office but I'm glad they do. It would be nice to have a representative whose sole job on the council was to represent and advocate for the older generation. I could envision the geriatric wing of City Hall.

Entry May 10
Freedom from Self-condemnation

Self-condemnation is almost self-explanatory but is much more gruesome than I originally thought. Self-condemnation is like the energizer bunny that kept on giving and giving. Positive criticism is welcome. It hurts but as long as it is constructive it is accepted. If someone has something unconstructive and negative to say about me and I took it in as true then it is the beginning of the end. Letting the negative thoughts in points me in a negative direction. Once inside and accepted by me they take root and the roller coaster of self-condemnation begins. If I took the same energy and accepted a positive statement and had it take root then I would be headed in a positive direction. Initially positive thoughts took longer for me to assimilate because I had so much negativity to weed. Somewhere I read it takes eight positive thoughts to change or reverse the direction of a single negative thought. I believe positive and negative thoughts have equal power. It is the predominant mind atmosphere of positive or negative that impacts the process. A positive thought in a positive thought environment could grow quickly. A negative thought in a positive thought environment could take longer to be sown if it could be sown at all. If the negative thought environment was pervasive it would kick out the positive thought. The reverse is true for a positive thought in a negative thought environment.

In retirement I have choices about the type of people I experience. At work my co-workers came with the job. My reaction to them was my choice. Now I can say no thank you and remove myself from any environment because my paycheck is not dependent upon it. Instead of being stuck I can say no thank you. "Being stuck" became my norm in my work life. I am now unstuck and have changed things to my liking. "Being stuck" thinking reincarnated into "I choose" or "I volunteer."

Self-condemnation is so painful because it brings up all related past hurts and old feelings of helplessness. I have more time to feel the feelings, which ultimately led to healing rather than repression. I reminded myself that repression was never a solution. But with self-condemnation the negative rippled long after the original insulters had exited the picture. And the person now condemning was I on myself. It was gruesome and there was no one to blame but me. The inner war did more damage than any verbal insult from a human. I remembered reading research about abuse. All abuse is horrible but emotional abuse without physical abuse is the worst. Physical abuse left visible evidence like bruises and broken bones in addition to the emotional aspect. Emotional abuse alone left no evidence; no bruises, no physical verification, only an unseen broken heart that could not be put in a cast. It is hard to know when the heart healed either way. The heart has to also heal after physical abuse but it was a known fact physical abuse broke the heart. Emotional abuse could fly below the radar and if unseen was probably unknown. It cannot be verified. Unseen emotional abuse included a hidden broken heart. Not being seen didn't stop the truth from being the truth. When healing occurred the poison no longer existed.

Everyone knows many examples of children whose parents were divorced. Some children internalize the blame and think the divorce was their fault. Without psychological help the child con-tinues to turn the guilt upon him or herself. It is another example of self-condemnation. What I wanted to practice was accepting other peoples' freedom to choose negativity without letting the negativity into my space. Everyone has free will and I couldn't change other people, only myself. If someone made a negative projection on me then I got angry. Calling them out could be a weakness. I wanted to right the situation and have them reel back their projection and accept it as theirs and not mine. Today there was a bombing in Jordan and yet I was more concerned about my own emotional body. I have no control over Jordan just as I have no control over other people and their thoughts. I wanted to know the line where other people's thoughts and words interfered with my ability to love. A wise person knows when to let the projections continue and when to say stop. With retirement I had the freedom to get out of any situation and the freedom to take care of myself. My goal was choosing wisely when self-condemnation reared its ugly head. Standing up for me is always wise. Using prayer to help me decide when was an option. If I am too emotional I just walk away until the emotions subside and I can see clearly.

Entry May 15
Personal Mission Statement

Almost everyone is familiar with the concept of a mission statement for a business or a non-profit organization. Many people are familiar with personal mission statements. I had done one for myself and have participated in assisting others when designing their own. A friend asked me to support her while she and some other people developed personal mission statements. I went and supported her. It made me wonder how powerful we are as individuals and how powerful we are when we support one another. Everyone in the group carried powerful words in his or her heart. Everyone defined words and meaning of words differently. Some had the same word but understood a different meaning for it. To support someone while she uncovered her personal energy behind words was fascinating and something I would highly recommend. It should be mandatory for retirees. Retirement is a life change with new goals. And thus, as a retiree, I had a new mission. It meant removing the blocks and old belief systems about retirement that interfered with my present moment. When I was twenty I would have defined retirement as stay at home and watch television because that was what my father did when he retired. His health was not particularly good so short infrequent walks were his activity. I had no idea how he felt about retirement because I never asked before he died. My projection onto him at that time was that he was bored. It wasn't until my fifties that I met people who were actively retired. Retirement was no longer synonymous with illness for me.

My mission statement was pursuing my passions while being active, healthy, and having fun. What I choose to do had to fit under the categories of my mission statement. It had to relate to my passions, being active, having fun, and/or being healthy. If not then I needed to choose again.

My personal word or mission statement became a safe place to go when faced with life's challenges. Another word for it was centering. Being centered kept the focus on wholesome, healthy thoughts and vibrations. No one could argue with the fact that words are powerful. It is best to use words for the positive or the productive in life. It was a positive to know the truth about how my thinking impacted my life.

Entry May 21
Freedom to Love

Love is illusive. Anyone who defines it restrains it. It can be manipulated to the point that it becomes anti love by virtue of manipulation. There are phrases that raised questions like "tough love," "I love ice cream," and "women who love too much." It breaks my heart to read about abused children who can't wait to get home to their abusive parents because they loved them. Sometimes a truth stays in my mind long after I read the words. This happened when I read God so loved his only son he sent him to earth to be crucified. Then there is the difference between loving one's self and loving others. The bottom line is, a person has to love himself before he can love another. Some of us treat other people as badly as we treat ourselves and wonder why we don't have any friends. Love can be felt. Being single and loving is perhaps like hearing one hand clap. It is easier to hear two hands clapping and feel two people living together loving each other. The answer lies within the question. Without sounding too religious there are Spirit or spirits who heard and hear everything. They hear beyond the human ear. I know I am free to experience every realm, every phrase. There are so many projections placed on a single never married heterosexual woman. I have concluded that love comes in all forms. Yet I believe I have reached a point where I can reflect on the projections and stand firm in who I am. The question isn't dealing with the judgments. It is dealing with acceptance or rejection of projections. If I truly know who I am then the projections are meaningless.

Entry May 31
Freedom to Age Healthy and With Grace

While working out at the YMCA I heard people comment, "once I turned fifty everything started to fall apart," "I feel worse which is natural since I turned sixty five," and "Don't get old." My response was "I feel better now at fifty seven than I did at forty seven." They looked at me as if I were nuts. It is great that I have retired and have the freedom to work out in my own time. I eat better because I can daily go to the store if I choose to. With freedom came responsibility and when it came to taking care of me physically I was doing that with food and exercise. It was a blessing to move through each day doing exactly what I wanted to do. There is the mundane like putting gas in the car or washing the car. It all seems so much lighter now that I didn't have the pressure of a job. The time squeeze was gone. I even had the freedom to be overwhelmed and decide to stay in bed all day if I chose to. That is freedom. There are consequences to every choice and every decision. It can be overwhelming. Food is a good example. If I eat a lot of fatty calories I gain weight. If I accept a lot of negative self-talk I create low self-esteem. It is so important to me to think of and thank every part of my body for everything it has done to keep me healthy. Had it been up to my senses I would not be healthy because I would have eaten what looked and tasted good. I don't know how to transform food into bones or skin but my body does. I groan when I think of what I put my feet through in any given day. These feet of mine have jogged on treadmills at the Club, hiked up the healing mountain in big heavy hiking boots, walked on sweaty floors when I went to Hot Yoga, danced with all my weight on them, and walked around the neighborhood. Wow that is loyalty. I have learned to be grateful.

While working out I talked to a friend about buying land or a ranch in the Show Low area. He looked shocked. He was dumbfounded and his comment was "neither you nor I will be alive in thirty years when it might be worth some money." My initial reaction was I wouldn't be buying it to make money. It would be for pleasure and being in the great outdoors. My secondary reaction was I'll be around forever; I'm not dying anytime soon. Thinking about my death wasn't something I wanted to give too much attention to. It was going to happen and while I accepted that, I intended to have fun before it knocked on my door. It is normal to deny death but denial isn't going to stop it from happening.

I remembered the first time I realized I was middle aged. It was a shock. In my life aging crept up. No pun intended. When Gloria Steinem turned forty, her response to a reporter telling her how great she looked was "what do you mean; this is what forty looks like."

The **Arizona Republic** on 11/28/05 had an article titled "Poll on Aging Reveal Fear of low life quality" by Anita Manning of **USA Today**. According to a **USA Today/ABC News** poll on aging "the idea of growing old apparently is scarier than growing old itself."

I concluded for myself that the idea of aging was scarier than the fact of aging. Ernest Holmes said, "Change your thinking, change your life." Now that was interesting. The article went on to discuss that people didn't think they could enjoy life as they approached one hundred years old. However, the poll also indicated that the older people get, the less worried they are about aging. It made me think that while I can't do anything about aging, I know I could do something about attitude. In the recesses of my mind I know that I have said I don't want to live if I can't feed myself, can't walk and can't bathe. Even today I saw a lady at Costco who looked so thin, so old, and she could barely walk. Yet there was a grace about her. It must be the difference in attitude. Just as I have the freedom to take better care of myself

I also know I am not twenty years old anymore. As long as I know I was taking care of me, I am okay.

The article went on "Many Americans have this idea that as you age, your health will decline and you will not be able to care for yourself. Younger people fear old age because of misconception that getting older means a rapid decline in health" says researcher JaeMi Pennington of the New England Centenarian Study at Boston University. "That's not necessarily so" Pennington says. "More people today are living longer and healthier lives, and we can attribute that to the advances in medical science and better nutrition".

My bones and body won't last forever but my soul was another matter. If any part of me was immortal then I came from somewhere and somewhere before that and so on. My body is a temporary temple. The better care I gave it, the longer it will last.

In another **Arizona Republic** article "Placebo effect helps in healing: study says" by Lauran Neegaard with the Associated Press states "Research is showing the power of expectations, that they have physical, not just psychological, effects on your health. Scientists can measure the resulting changes in the brain, from the release of natural painkilling chemicals to alterations in how neurons fire. Among the most provocative findings: New research suggest that once Alzheimer's disease robs someone of the ability to expect that a proven painkiller will help them, it doesn't work nearly as well".

The role my expectations will play in my aging process is yet to be determined. I keep finding shards, like the articles above, along the way.

My garden is just perfect in the early morning sun. Everything is bearing fruit or blossoming. Weeds were pulled and the water bubbling system made a trickling sound that drew birds. I sip my coffee knowing this was the time to relax and enjoy the labors of a well-planned garden. The garden reflected my retirement.

Section II
The Present or the
Beginning

Chapter 1

Thunderbird Mountain

With all my newfound insights I sensed my maturity and thought I was pretty cool. Hiking had become a real passion. Earlier in the summer three rattlesnakes and a swarm of bees on the trail at Thunderbird Mountain had challenged me. With cooler weather in Phoenix my urge to hike the mountain was greater than any fears of snakes and bees. I called a couple of friends but no one was game to hike. So I went alone. It was chilly sweater weather in the fifties, which was cold for Phoenix. My first vocal thought as I drove to the mountain was "I hope the snakes are hibernating." Channel twelve news warned hikers to be cautious of rattlers that were still feeding off the land before hibernation. There were no good hiding places for snakes on the dusty, rocky trails this time of year. No brush to hide them. Last spring the mountain was green and lush with shrubbery and wildflowers that hid snakes quite well. When summer sun hit and temperatures soared above one hundred, everything turned brown, died, and blew away. The trail would be pretty stark with only rocks for hiding spaces.

It was a glorious day with a sizeable crowd if I counted all the cars in the parking lot. I tucked my water and apple into my fanny pack and realized I had left my cell phone at home. Perhaps it was false security but having my cell phone within reach made me more comfortable on lone hikes. 911 was a dial away. With hiking stick in hand I began the uphill trek and it was all familiar. I sensed the mountain welcoming me back with open arms. The sun wasn't too hot and there was a breeze, thank God. It was fairly late in the day and I didn't expect to see any regulars because of the late hour. My regular group came earlier in the day generally between eight and nine am. Several people were on the trail but none who I knew. It was a short two-mile hike and, what a relief, I didn't have to deal with snakes or bees. When I returned home after hiking solo that afternoon I relaxed in an Epsom salt bath. After my bath I focused in my bathroom mirror and lazily fingered through my newly permed curly hair. I swear my eyes twinkled. I kept a steady gaze for a few minutes and attributed the twinkle to my reunion with the healing mountain.

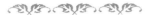

Several days later I took the full hike, which was close to four miles. As I rounded the last switchback my eyes came upon Jareed and his dog, Shade. They were headed up the mountain. I waited for him to be within ear shot and shouted.

"Hi, how was summer?" He responded with a wave. I could see Jareed lean over his dog.

"Look Shade there is a familiar face."

Shade wagged his tail but, as usual, remained behind his master. I recollected my first conversation last year with Jareed when it was a hundred and five degrees. Back then I didn't see any bottles of water on Jareed so I offered him one of my extra bottles for his dog. I remember Jareed's look of surprise and irritation at my question.

"My dog doesn't need to drink water on the mountain."

I, of course, had trouble accepting that bit of information.

"Dogs have fur coats and need water."

I insisted but Jareed corrected me.

"Look we are from Arabia and Americans drink too much water."

We both chuckled. I wondered if Jareed remembered that conversation from last year. I had gone on and on about how dogs died on Squaw Peak (now Piestewa Peak) from dehydration. Careless owners neglected to bring water for their dogs. As a result dogs were no longer allowed on Squaw Peak. I was happy for the dogs. Every year when the temperature dropped into the eighties I was relieved because less water was needed in the cooler temperatures.

Jareed and Shade walked in front of me and I was glad to see someone from my past. It made my heart feel good. There used to be a dozen regulars on the mountain. Many, including myself, skipped climbing in the hotter summer months.

"How was your summer, Nancy? Have you saved any dogs?"

We both laughed, pleased that our conversation from last year was remembered. After some small talk Jareed and Shade continued on their uphill hike and I returned my focus to a downhill return to the parking lot.

The trail made a four-mile loop around the mountain with the mid point being the top so a person could come from either direction and meet in the middle. My favorite route was the east side up and down. The view was better. I was drawn to the horses and students who rode at the riding school below that mountain. Just above the one-mile marker the horses would come into view.

Some days I heard horses before I saw them. Their beauty and form was breathtaking and reminded me that Phoenix was still part of the old west. But, on that day I observed the riding school was gone; lock, stock, and barrel. Aside from two large crop circles that looked like the old arenas nothing was left. I made a mental note to ask one of the regular hikers what had happened and when the school had left. All the little things that reminded me of the Wild West were disappearing. I couldn't remember the last time I saw a person riding a horse through the Jack in the Box drive-through window to order a soda. It was now common for horse properties to be sold for a lot of money; the land was valuable and needed for development. That which made Phoenix so great to me was being replaced with development. It saddened me to see natural settings disappear. Nature, however, always has the last word, it will resurrect and the horse property will pop up somewhere else, probably not within my sight. The healing properties of the mountain aren't dependent on the horse stables.

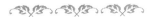

The next day instead of hiking I went to the YMCA. It was too hot to hike. My neighbor, Gina, from down the street, had renamed the YMCA "The Club." Gina and I had many laughs as we discussed The Club and its members. One man at The Club had his eye on Gina and he was quickly nicknamed Gina's crush. Nothing came of the attraction. As Gina put it "you never know about someone: if it was meant to be nature would take its course." I, however, believe nature sometimes needed a shove.

As the days got cooler my frequency to The Club decreased. The Club was convenient, about a five-minute drive. The healing mountain was a thirty-minute drive. Given the availability of time for an hour round trip drive I generally selected my healing mountain.

It was no surprise that the following week at eight in the morning my day started on the trail. From the bottom, looking up, the mountain resembled a pile of rocks and dirt with four peaks that reached a mile into the sky. The mountain trail wound its way into invisibility on the left and seemed to reappear on the upper bend in the mountain. There were trees like Palo Verde and Mesquite that were more like big bushes compared to the pine trees up north. As a child my thoughts of desert and Phoenix were of a sand desert with only brown sand. Living here I had learned desert bushes turn green and some do flower and yet the tumbleweed would get so dry, it would blow away. The desert had seasons. The desert brush today was brown and barren. As I started down the trail I saw Ted headed up. He used to wear a bright orange shirt that made him visible a mile away. He always had an earphone plugged in his ear as he listened intently to music or a book. His eyes would be focused on the trail. That day I saw him long before he saw me. Last time I saw him his hand was injured and bandaged. He said he was fine and we had planned to meet the following morning at ten for a hike together. Next day I arrived by ten but no Ted. Our standing agreement for meeting at the mountain was to wait ten minutes for the other, then hike without him. We never exchanged phone numbers so there was no way to follow up. I assumed his hand injury altered our plan to hike. He probably forgot because the subject never came up. Mountain conversations are non-intrusive and without judgment. Talk if you want and don't if you choose not to. People hike to feel good and a bunch of unsolicited questions could border on analysis. It flattens the freedom of just being. Although I wouldn't recommend this type of relationship in negotiating a contract or doing business, there is a peace in being present in the moment on the mountain. It is less risky to share with some indirect person not in your daily world.

What surprised me most as I observed Ted head toward me was he was wearing dark navy blue instead of bright orange. I was relieved to see a bright yellow water bottle hanging from his fanny pack.

"Hey Ted, how the heck are you?" He looked up in total surprise and turned his CD player to off.

"How was your summer, Nancy?"

"Hot, I was in Phoenix for most of it." He chuckled and told me about his trip to Alaska for his granddaughter's wedding. I couldn't tell if it was a teardrop or a bead of perspiration on his cheek. I remembered past personal mountain conversations; the kinds that were so honest that my heart split open like a seed. Pure honesty is beautiful. When someone gets to the core of either a positive or a negative emotion the truth of it reverberates through me. It takes courage to rip off masks and let sunlight into the dark corners. Nothing is more elegant than feeling truth.

"What happened to the horses and the riding school?"

Ted accepted my change of subject.

"I watched all summer; they slowly and painstakingly removed each piece of lumber and whatever else had to be removed from all the stalls. All that was left by the end of August was bare ground. See the large rectangular areas, that's where the horse stalls were, remember? And the huge circles over there where the horses were ridden, gone. I heard the riding school got kicked out because the land became too valuable for just horses. It was sold to developers and now we get to watch houses being built. Watching houses being built is better than watching horses play in the fields don't you think Nancy?"

"Like going to a dentist." It felt good to see Ted. It wouldn't have been okay if I had never seen him again. We were mountain friends.

"How is retirement going? Any regrets? I know you were concerned about money, are you working or fully retired?"

"It is better than I ever could have imagined. I think my anxiety was about entering something new, you know, unknown. Once I settled down it all fell in place with the money."

"I told you, you spend less. Emotionally how are you doing?"

"I've never been better. It is like someone took a ninety-pound weight off my shoulders. I didn't realize how stressed I was and for how long. Literally it was like someone sucked negative energy out of me. It had to come out and I am so much lighter, not to mention thinner. Truthfully I lost weight; I think I used to eat to comfort myself."

"You had to listen to a lot of problems, how could you not pick up that energy?"

"Secondary stress came with the job but it wasn't from clients, it was more from the politics of the working environment. I see it so clearly now that I am gone. Now it is like a past dream with no impact. Some people tell me I glow I am so happy."

"I always thought you glowed, you are a good person." The affirmation coming from Ted tickled me. It was a good thing we were standing still or I might have tripped. Lots of rocks all sizes cover this trail. It was a balancing act to not trip while hiking and looking at views.

"Thanks, sometimes I wonder what took me so long to leap into retirement. It was one of my best decisions. It all worked out.

Thanks for asking. Verbalizing it makes me more aware and feels safer. No extra job needed yet, thank God. I'm cool cleaning and clearing out."

"I'm so glad. You deserve it; I'll listen to you any time. You would have done it for me. Hey, I must get going. See you later this week?"

"Yeah." I extended my hand and tried to see his eyes through the dark sunglasses. Ted grabbed my hand with both of his. Eyes are the mirrors of the soul I've heard. I wanted to see his soul. When someone is happy his or her eyes sparkle and I was happy to see him. I wanted to see in his eyes that he was happy to see me.

"Come on give me a hug."

Yes, we were mountain friends. I liked Ted. He was open and communicated his feelings well. I concluded he felt safe with me because I wasn't part of his day-to-day life. Ted stood about six feet tall with a stocky build. His long hair and beard were salt and pepper. His grin reached from ear to ear. As best as I could guess he was about sixty years old. I knew he was married for a second time and retired and that was about all I knew of him.

Before I reached the bottom of the mountain I came upon Stan. Stan had been in Michigan with his huge family for the summer.

"Hey Nancy," he roared. He was a big guy, who had retired from Ford Motor Company several years ago and moved to Arizona. Stan and I both observed rattle snakes on the trail last year. Stan had raised the question to me.

"Why do we hike with so many snakes?" The word snakes made the hair on my neck stand up.

"There is risk in most things; we must love hiking this mountain."

The month of May was when baby snakes became visible and slithered on the trails. The snakes claimed their home as the mountain. Last year I had also discussed the possible purchase of a new Subaru. Stan had objections.

"Subaru is not American made. Don't you care?"

He was right. He talked about the working conditions in some of the foreign countries where the workers in the manufacturing plants had fifteen hour days, six days a week, with no recognition of overtime.

"Americans earn and are paid for their overtime. In the foreign plants overtime is not paid but the workers are required to work it for free. Is that what you want to support Nancy?"

"No wonder overseas factories can sell their cars cheaper."

Stan knew I had heard him and, of course, I stopped consideration of a Subaru. It was another benefit of friends and conversations on the mountain. We had stepped off the trail to let a couple of other hikers with their dog pass. Both Stan and I watched them as they tripped over rocks trying to go fast. Everybody was in a hurry to get to the top. The mountaintop from the bottom looks like Mount Everest. Stan stepped back on the trail to continue his hike. I had one last question.

"Stan did you eat Kielbasa sausage back in Michigan?"

He grinned from ear to ear.

"Yes but I am more glad to be back hiking this mountain. Good to see you Nancy." And he was up the trail.

"Bye." I stood a minute and watched him ascend. He had a good, steady pace.

I neared the end of my four miles and turned the final bend. Before me were flashing red lights in the parking lot. I could not imagine what on earth could be going on. I knew for certain it wasn't a church group passing out water bottles. I could see my chili pepper red Jeep Cherokee and, thank God, no one was around it. As I got closer to the parking lot I saw someone's car window was shattered and the police were dusting for prints. In the parking lot one of the cops explained the problem to me.

"There has been a rash of thieves breaking car windows and grabbing wallets or purses in this parking lot. The thieves know they have to work fast because people are always coming and going to the mountain. It is a short window of opportunity for a thief."

The car, with two broken windows, was two parking slots away from my car. I offered my sympathy to the car owners and was glad no valuables had been stolen. I decided to put a sign in my car window "no valuables inside." It would probably be more of an amusement than a deterrent.

I opened the hatch on the back of my jeep and retrieved another bottle of water as I changed out of my hiking boots. I was disappointed I hadn't seen more of the regular hikers but I saw the ones I was closest to, my mountain friends. My hopes were heightened; in the next few weeks perhaps I would see them all.

Chapter 2

Red Rock Country

George and I planned to meet at a predetermined location, Anthem Outlet Mall, at nine on a Tuesday morning. Meeting at Anthem Outlet Mall worked out best for our hiking trips up north. Anthem Mall was on the way to our destination, Sedona. In considering this hiking friend I often thought it was too bad we weren't physically attracted to one another. Dating was never an option as George was gay. We had worked together for many years and now both of us were retired and into hiking. He was sixty-five and looked forty-five. He was into fashion with his hair always perfect and his clothes stylish. He lived far west of Phoenix and I was in the central corridor. On our scheduled morning he got a late start and called me around eight in the morning.

"I'm late and have to stop for gas but I will be there."

I was in the middle of making a peanut butter and jelly sandwich for the hike and managed to smear the phone with peanut butter. I was very appreciative of George's thoughtfulness.

"Not everyone is so considerate."

"You say that and yet you are probably pissed, you are always on time." He was right I liked being on time. Other people being late, here and there, was okay with me, especially if they called to let me know. Habitually late people don't show up in my world.

"Just get there safely okay?"

I beat him to the mall. Once we were together I grabbed my stuff and threw it in the back of his SUV and we were off. The whole way to Sedona we both talked about how happy we were to be free and retired. He incessantly chewed gum. It was an observation not worth any conversation. It would have bothered me in a quiet room. Here in a car with music, and my good friend, nothing bothered me. For something to bother me I have to give it permission. It wasn't going to happen today.

"While everybody else is working away we are on the road to Sedona, isn't it great?" George savored the freedom to do whatever he wanted. He and I understood that kind of freedom.

"No hurry, just relaxing in luxury while you drive."

"It is an attitude of relaxation, we got it made don't you think?" George is right about attitude. When my attitude is healthy everything else falls into place. The attitude creates more of itself. If my attitude is bad then it will multiply and creates more negativity.

"You can sleep Nancy if you want while I drive."

Riding in a car always made me sleepy. Old friends are like old slippers, they are comfortable and know you. I liked that he knew little things about me.

"Wake me if you want me to drive."

"Deal."

Sedona was about an hour and half drive from Phoenix. It is the most beautiful red rock country that one could imagine. I woke up as George made the turn off the freeway. The red mountains were in the far distance. George noticed my movement.

"It is always breathtaking."

"Keep you eyes on the road, George." It was a gentle reminder couched in a teasing tone. George was a safe driver. We both were quiet as he drove into town.

"It is like being in church, Nancy."

We passed Bell Rock and Cathedral Rock. The looming red rock formations were named; many of the names represented what the rock looked like; Bell Rock like a four story bell by the side of the road and Cathedral Rock like a church building. The road twisted and turned and of course ahead was an outlet mall. We zipped past it.

"Where's the ranger station? I need a bathroom break after driving up here, while you slept, young lady."

"Make me feel bad, it's in that center on the left, we can check with the rangers on conditions around Boynton."

"And buy a day pass."

"Good by me I'll pay since you drove."

"It looks like a perfect day." We both shifted our weight around in our seats. I pulled on my seat belt and stretched my legs against the floorboard. George moved his head from side to side. He parked, the car doors opened and we spilled out heading for the bathrooms.

After the bathroom break we perused the travel area and decided we were good to go with no problems noted in Boynton Canyon. After a fifteen-minute drive we arrived at the parking lot and pulled into the last parking place. We were surprised at the crowd because it was a Tuesday morning. George lowered his designer sunglasses.

"Don't they know this is for us retired people?" He made me laugh. He had a great sense of humor and could find humor in the simplest things. We laughed a lot when we were together.

"Tell them George."

We changed into hiking boots and headed for the trail. The trailhead was five hundred feet straight ahead. The trail appeared to run parallel to the fence that enclosed the exclusive Enchantment Resort. The Resort was a "top of the line luxury" resort.

"You ever read any newspaper articles about this resort blocking Indians from getting to their sacred grounds in the canyon?"

The resort had opened in 2000 and supposedly blocked anyone from entering the canyon, which was Native American sacred land. The Indians protested.

"I read something awhile back; they must have decided to open it up."

"I'm glad."

With hiking sticks in hand we began the adventure. The old brittle leaves crunched under our boots. Leaves that had fallen created a blanket of yellow, red, orange, and brown of various shades that covered the trailhead. The coolness in the air felt like heaven. George unbuttoned his jacket.

"Don't need jackets in this piece of heaven."

Enormous trees shaded the start of the trail. Big boulders of red clay were visible all around us. The color contrasted to the desert brown of Thunderbird Mountain. The silence other than our footsteps was eerie. Patches of what looked like forests of trees loomed in the distance. George broke the silence.

"This is mystical man, in the eighties people hiked vortexes in Sedona for energy. You hear about that?"

"Yeah and I was one of them."

"Well then, young lady, you supposedly know that there are three high energy points on the planet; Sussex, England; the Bermuda Triangle off the Florida coast; and Sedona, Arizona. Vortexes are electric, magnetic, or some combination. A vortex with both electric and magnetic energy is the most powerful. Boynton Canyon is supposedly that. It is the one and only vortex with both electric and magnetic energy. It compares to a masculine and a feminine energy. Did you know that? You believe it?"

George surprised me. His realm of knowledge covered a wide spectrum. We were literally steeped in this vortex energy. I felt something but it was hard to distinguish if it was the vortex or my senses absorbing nature. I get the same feeling when I walk in a woods, watch a sunset, or hike my healing mountain.

"In the beginning I questioned it, it seemed like a marketing tool but then I had my own experiences. The flip side is I was susceptible to suggestion. What matters was I felt something. There have been too many testimonials for me to negate the power."

"How do you know all that? You believe it or just read about it."

George tended to see the glass half empty especially if he is in a bad mood. With retirement his mood has been consistently up. He has been more exploratory and more fun.

"I hiked here a lot in the eighties and heard some crazy stuff. No personal experience. Anything that is good and positive is good with me. Real or not I don't care if it makes people feel better." I surmised he thought it was crazy but it worked to make people happy. I chose to believe there was more of a real cause to the effect.

"I like the feminine energy part. Never quite thought of it that way. Makes me think the feminine is the magnetic and the masculine the electric. Is that true? "

"I can't remember back that far, but it sounds logical."

"We can meditate when we get to the top and reach our own conclusions."

"You are an old feminist, female power and all that stuff." I loved George; he had no filters and said whatever was on his mind. It surprised me that he knew more than I about the vortexes. He never struck me as being philosophical.

We rounded the corner and looked up at small resort casitas. The iron fence bordering the walkway made it clear that no trespassing onto the resort was allowed. There was even a sign on the fence, advising people that the fence was under electronic surveillance 24/7.

George was first to react. "How sad all this man made crap."

We had passed several people and each time we exchanged verbal niceties. After passing what felt like the twentieth casita I stopped a hiker headed to the parking lot.

"Are the casitas ever going to end? Is there a point when this resort ends and we are in the woods?"

The hiker chuckled. Behind us were a row of casitas and a forest of trees interspersed with tall pointy roofs. I wasn't sure which looked more surreal; the red boulders growing up out of the lush forest or the concrete castle tops poking their heads out of the forest. It had to be perception. He pointed in the direction George and I were hiking.

"Yes, see the brown smoke stack just ahead."

"Yes." George chimed in.

"That is the last sign of civilization on the path. You will then be entering the quietness of the canyon."

"Thank God." And on we went.

Every turn on the path was more beautiful than the last. The trail meandered through a creek that was running with water. Arizona is full of dry creek beds especially in summer. The beds dry up and when monsoon season hits the rains fill a dry bed in a matter of minutes. People have drowned because of the quick and unexpected flow of raging water. Campers knew better than to pitch a tent in a dry creek bed.

The smells were pine and cedar mixed with fresh air. Rocks were in all sizes and the only ones I dreaded were the tiny ones that snuck in my boot. It became quieter and more peaceful the farther we progressed along the path. Red rocks jutted out in primitive formations, some taller than a four-story building. Falling leaves floated through the air. It was surreal. I imagined a tree nymph like the one I had painted in art class winking at us from behind each tree. When the sun shone through the branches it was mystical. Everything twinkled. Every so often people came down from the top and each time I noted the peace and the shine in their eyes. It is one thing to talk about peace but to experience that peace unfolding in the eyes of strangers thrilled me. It humbled me to be in a place of such awakening.

"Nancy, are you getting hungry yet?"

George keeps me in physical reality. "Food always sounds good to me."

We found the next fallen tree limb, sat down, and began eating. Lunch was spent mostly in silence interspersed with small talk. In between chews and speaking George passed me some granola.

"I love being with old friends, I don't have to impress or entertain you."

I liked the fact that George was so relaxed with me; no airs, he could be himself. It was that feeling for me of being at home in my old slippers. Like I felt on the car ride up here, I can just be me.

"You say that because I am a woman, just kidding, I know what you mean. We are comfortable in our skins. I love spending time with you; there is no judgment, just hiking and peace."

"And a few bad jokes. It's interesting the way you put it, you know sometimes you see couples and they don't talk and they look bored. We don't talk and it is okay. I wonder if someone observing us would think otherwise, perhaps that we are bored?"

"I doubt it because our eyes are taking it all in, you know, like occupied and stimulated."

"Not crazy stimulated but peacefully engaged. Yeah girl we got it."

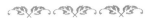

After lunch we continued our elevation through the canyon to the top. The last part of the hike before the top included scaling large boulders the size of a small planet. When we got to the base of the boulder area we met two ladies with heavy Boston accents. The ladies were quiet, sitting on individual tree stumps enjoying their lunch. One of them put her sandwich down.

"Ahoy there, and welcome." George was ahead of me so he addressed them first.

"Hello and welcome to you too, you are from Boston I take it."

They both nodded. "And we are Red Sox fans."

"And we are Arizona fans."

One of the Boston ladies quickly named the ledge they were sitting on.

"This is *The Café* with no waiters, it's a bring your own kind of place, have a seat."

I sat.

"Are you on vacation?" I brushed off red clay dust from my hiking pants and pulled up a rock.

"I'm Jan and this is Judy; our husbands are up ahead, we got tired and shooed them on."

"Are you sure they will be back?" George couldn't help himself.

"We would rather talk to some regulars from Phoenix."

George winked at us and continued his climb, ignoring their invitation.

"I'm Nancy. Just excuse him; he is on a mission to reach the top. This is only our second hike together in Sedona; we both just retired and decided to have a fun day.

"George I'll catch up." I turned back to the ladies. "We're driving back to Phoenix after our hike. He wants to reach the top and be back at the car by dark. The canyon here gets dark very early; the sun can't shine through the trees to light the trail through the deep canyon. Remember all those twist and turns, when you just see rocks and more rocks? Don't get stuck either."

The ladies leaned back against the rocks, each getting comfortable. They didn't appear to be in a hurry and were un-phased. They reminded me of good ole girls with a story to tell. Some came to Sedona to search for beauty and some for spirituality.

"Jan and I are new retirees also; our husbands have been retired for years."

"Were you afraid at all to retire? I'm single so it was a leap for me."

"For me no, Jan can answer for herself. I'm sixty-five and my office had a hard rule of automatic retirement at sixty-five. Jack, my husband, kept collecting all this travel information and I thought let's go. We've been to Florida, California, and next month to Italy. It's great and I have never looked back."

Jan looked at Judy who had just swallowed the last of her sandwich.

"My husband is a cancer survivor and well, our time is precious. Neither of us had pensions like Jack and Judy but our dividends are good. We even thought about buying a motor home but gas is so expensive."

I was grateful for how willing they were to share. "Emotionally how did each of you feel that first morning of retirement?"

Judy was quick and Jan was contemplative.

"It felt awkward that first day, our entire married life we had both worked and now we will both be home together virtually all of the time. It was like remembering who this man was when we first met, it was all good but different. As far as co-workers no real after-thoughts or emotions, we all meet periodically for lunch but that will fade out over time. You know I was a secretary at a law firm, which was not exactly a warm and fuzzy place to work. So far so good, retirement was a good decision."

We all shifted our position sitting among the rocks. Three sets of eyes soaking in the view while nibbling. We must have looked like three ladybugs sitting on rocks. A breeze blew through and surrounded us with a pine scent. I felt like I was in a western movie; sitting in the middle of nowhere with a couple of strangers just talking. Jan broke the silence.

"Ralph, my hubby, was getting chemo so my experience was different. I had taught for years and my insurance carried us. His cancer was like a cloud over everything, and I think my work was an escape for me. I would never tell Ralph that. I miss getting dressed up for work. I only started working ten years ago. That was when he got his diagnosis and the prospect of medical bills overwhelmed us. I went back to work. Now he is in remission. Not a day goes by that I don't give thanks for our day together."

"They have a real love story. Are you two married?" Judy stood as she spoke and stretched her legs. Her body faced me. These were ladies I would like to know better in Phoenix and yet there was this familiar feeling of mountain people and hiking on my healing mountain. Had I met them at a party our conversation would probably have been different and superficial.

"This is only your second hike with him right?" I nodded yes.

"Being single with one paycheck makes a difference. Honestly I was scared. I was only fifty-five and it seemed so final to be retired. Now I love it. The money seems to work out; I spend less on clothes, gas, parking, and food. Most of all I am free."

Strange male voices, obviously the aforementioned husbands, Jack and Ralph, were getting louder as they came from behind a huge boulder.

"You girls still there?" It must have been Jack talking because Judy responded first.

"We didn't run. Did you see a lone man hiking up there?"

"You mean George? Yes, we met."

"This is Nancy, they just retired and are up here celebrating their freedom."

Jan was right on. I smiled and shook hands with Ralph and Jack. Ralph was very thin but his eyes sparkled.

"You both have that Sedona glaze in your eyes. It is beautiful up here isn't it?"

Ralph raised his hand with palm facing the sun.

"This is God's country."

I picked up my stick. "I better find George, he could leave me here. Enjoy."

The Boston ladies grinned and Judy raised a pointed finger at me.

"Have fun in retirement, life is short."

"Nice to meet you folks, enjoy Sedona." It was a genuine conversation; in nature I concluded people talked about anything. One thing was for sure, I was glad I was retired.

It mesmerized me when I grabbed hold of a red rock. They were powdery and solid at the same time. I was alone and immersed in a rainbow of red and green vapor. The wind blew and visions of red clouds hovered over a sea of green trees. The formations of huge rock proportions invited me to climb and as I got higher and higher I realized I was looking down on the trees.

What loomed large over me in the beginning of the hike now was beneath me. The view from the top of the canyon was a green river of trees flowing through a red canyon of rocks. After a lot of my loud grunts I reached the top and heard George.

"It's about time you got here."

The view was spectacular. "Can you believe this beauty?"

"This is Arizona Nancy, how did we get so lucky to live here? Now if we could just liberalize people and get them to vote democratic."

"Too funny."

We laughed, joked, and even meditated for an hour. We concluded the energy was both masculine and feminine. Equal opportunity. We were both grateful. George looked at his watch.

"Hey it's four, ready to go?"

"Do you always bear such good news? I know it's a drive back, let's go?"

On the way down I noticed George picking up leaves that he then tucked in his backpack.

"What are you doing with the leaves?"

"These." He pulled some out to show me. "I want to decorate my family room in these colors." They were an array of colors. He was anxious to complete the redecorating prior to his family visiting from Germany. George was born in Germany and had moved to Phoenix as a baby. Most of his mother's family still lived in Germany. We continued down the path stopping for special views and water breaks. It was about six and dark when we reached the car. I was tired and glad to remove my hiking boots and I could see that George felt the same. My sandals were in the car and felt great on my feet. We crunched on apples as we relaxed on the hood of the car. I heard a strange sound; like a dog crying as we downed cold drinks. I scanned the area and tried to figure the source of the sound. George ignored it and continued crunching without interruption. I slid off the hood and poked my hiking stick in the bushes just to make a sound.

"George what is that sound?" He didn't know. Then a coyote slyly crossed in front of us.

"Holy Shit." George spoke quietly.

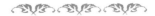

It was after eight when we reached Phoenix. We said our goodbyes. Thanksgiving was coming up and George wasn't sure if he could hike or meet again this month. He was leaving town to visit his daughter and her family in California.

"Nancy we will talk and get together if not before when I get back from California. Are you staying in town for the holiday?"

"Yes and will probably have a neighborhood thing in my yard, who knows."

"One of these years I am coming to your hood." We hugged.

Chapter 3

Thunderbird Mountain Didn't Change; I Did

I awoke to the sound of raindrops, which was considered miraculous during our draught. It hadn't rained in weeks. I could hardly wait to get to the mountain so I could hike in the rain. Weather in Phoenix changed rapidly. I could handle rain today with my lightweight rain jacket rolled up in my fanny pack along with a bottle of water, cell phone, lip balm, and an apple. By the time I parked at the mountain and got out of the car the rain had stopped. Coolness and moisture remained and I smelled the rain. It was cool for Phoenix probably seventy-five degrees. I began my familiar trek. The breeze was blowing stronger and I thought it doesn't get any better. I felt so lucky to live in America and to be so healthy.

This time on the mountain I ran into Sue. Sue was a regular and, like me, was just getting back into the routine of regular hiking. The only regular hiker through the summer was Ted. I didn't want to imagine what it was like hiking in 115° weather with snakes and other desert creatures. I imagined Ted with his earphones and brightly colored clothing going about his hike as if nothing else was going on. It was not something I would do but he enjoyed it. He was oblivious to his surroundings. I wanted to hear everything. I don't like animal surprises on the mountain.

Sue talked about her summer. "I had a marvelous summer. I went to Austria and did a lot in the great outdoors. Have you ever been to Austria, Nancy?"

"Yes and I got lost for about three hours. I learned a lot about me in that lost time."

Sue lifted her long narrow stick and motioned toward me. "I ordered new hiking sticks or I guess you call them trekking sticks. They were on sale; two for seventy dollars. Do you think that was a good deal?"

"My sticks were seventy dollars a piece from the Hiking Shack. I purchased two but I am most comfortable using only one. One gives me balance; two sticks and I trip over myself."

"I ordered a pair because I am tired of carrying this big, long stick. It gets heavy and then I fell last week and the damn stick didn't help at all."

"Are you okay?"

"Yeah I am fine but I have a bruised ego."

The rain had left large puddles on the path. I gestured in front of me.

"It is refreshing and muddy."

Sue side stepped the puddle, waved and went on ahead at her usual faster clip. She left me in the dust.

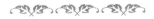

My mind floated and thoughts of proper hiking etiquette entertained me as I hiked. The person headed up the trail toward the top has the right of way. The person descending steps aside to let the ascender continue his trek up hill. It didn't matter much because most places on the trail were wide enough for two people to pass. I played interesting scenarios in my mind about polite and rude people. Some might just barrel through like a train and others maybe were polite and courteous. I chuckled to myself; it was just like life, I concluded. As a retiree, I was never in a hurry. Just let them pass.

Last year someone ran downhill and almost knocked George over into un-forgiving rocks. George, as a habit, stepped aside for anyone coming up or down, he was polite. Not me, the old me had to be right. I knew I had a stubborn streak. As long as there was room for two people I continued and didn't stop. If I was the ascender I continued. If I was descending then I stepped aside. I justified not stopping while ascending because it was hard to stop uphill on steep switchbacks. Momentum was more energetic going uphill. It was easier to stop when going downhill. That was the truth according to me. Now I just let them pass. The thought of anyone falling into rocks cured my need to be right.

When I got to the parking lot at the bottom there seemed to be a dozen people in a circle talking. My first thought was another car break in but there were no cops or red lights. I reached bottom, crossed the street into the parking lot and saw Sue in the circle. She motioned me to join.

"A reporter is here to interview us."

That was weird I thought and it probably has nothing to do with me. It did however, peak my curiosity.

"Why is he interviewing us in a parking lot? If it's about the mountain he needs to be at the top, the story is at the top."

The reporter, John, overheard my comment. "Not enough time. Why do people climb and continue to climb the same mountain?"

I thought he was suggesting it could get boring. "Have you ever climbed here?"

"Yes many years ago."

Amusing. It must have been a slow day at the newspaper. I liked his straightforwardness. He threw out questions and listened intently as each person responded. Some walked away after a couple of minutes but Sue and I stayed. Everyone pontificated on the beauty of the mountain and all the related health benefits of hiking. John seemed to like the flow of conversation. It was all positive, but it didn't feel real. The story to me was the hike itself.

"Tell me about the regulars up here on the mountain, the regular hikers?"

Several names were thrown out and he wrote them on his pad.

"When is the best time for pictures of the regulars and, of course, the best time for the regulars?"

I was hesitant. Mostly I liked privacy. Erosion was impacted negatively by large numbers of people hiking. "We don't want to increase the mountain population."

"It is just a story on hiking; look I will hike with you guys to the top for pictures and if people prefer I'll only shoot the back of their heads if they don't want their face in it. Is that good?"

Everyone was happy. I didn't care because I wasn't ready to commit to going.

"Okay, then I will be here next Thursday morning with a photographer around ten on top of the mountain. Whoever is there is there."

Five of us remained and we all shook John's hand. I wasn't going to participate in the photo. Photography had been a hobby of mine. I preferred to be behind the camera, not in front of it.

Retirement had so many benefits. When I worked it was mandatory to appear on television and radio shows to discuss youth programs. I considered myself a private person and, given choice, I wouldn't want to appear in any media. As a retiree I had choices. I was happy about choice. Sue, on the other hand, was excited about showcasing the mountain and was definitely planning on having her picture taken. That was the freedom of choice.

The other three people who I barely knew indicated they would be there with Sue. John was sure the photographer would like the assignment of climbing a mountain and it was as good as done.

I didn't like the thought of my quiet mountain turned into a tourist spot. This was Phoenix and it wouldn't be the first time things had changed as a result of a newspaper story. More people would come and more parking spaces would be needed. Hiking was a healthy choice but all I wanted was not to have a crowd on this mountain.

Chapter 4

Always a Family

When I returned home my phone was ringing as I opened the door. It was my sister-in- law. I had expected her call. My brother had been scheduled for knee surgery on this day. Last year he had successful hip surgery. He was in my prayers and thoughts. Surgery helps to heal and was drastic at the same time. Hiking my mountain and praying kept me in the present and out of worry. Hiking was how I coped. Worrying does nothing. Worrying and praying are mutually exclusive.

"Your brother is fine; he came through his knee surgery with flying colors."

"Great. You don't sound so good." I was relieved but not surprised. My brother has a strong constitution. I could hear the raspy tones in my sister-in-law's voice. The caretaker sometimes gets lost in the shuffle. The stress of the day was hitting her.

She had no complaints about my brother today.

Millie, my sister-in-law, had the flu. Tom and Millie had been married for thirty-five years and for most of those thirty-five years Millie had complained. I thought she liked to complain because she did a lot of it. She was always divorcing my brother. He wasn't perfect. He, like me, combined the best of the Irish and the best of the German. We could drink and we could work. He was approaching sixty. Last year he became the proud recipient of new hips. Not one hip at a time as most regular folks would do. He had both hips done. That way he only had to pay the deductible one time. They don't call Notre Dame the Fighting Irish for nothing. Tom could attest to that. He had graduated from there. My brother and I were raised in a small Kentucky town, famous for both its Irish and German heritage. Our father had worked in the post office and our mother in a bakery. We lived in a rural area with cows and a garden. The work ethic was strong. My father went to work no matter what. He died at work with a heart attack. My mother died in her sleep, as she wanted. She wasn't sick for very long. My brother and I were with her. It was peaceful.

We lived across the country from each other but I always felt closeness as they did. Family was an interesting dynamic; if we lived closer Millie would probably complain about me too. It was her way or maybe I had become a safe place to dump her negativity. Either way I saw through her. I wished she would see that her negativity created more.

I said good-bye to Millie on the phone and wished her pleasant dreams and better health in the morning. I hung up and immediately called Tom in the hospital. I knew he would be a doctor's idea of a perfect patient. He was strong and independent. He answered the phone.

"Hi Nancy, I just got back from walking down the hall. The knee surgery was successful."

He talked away about the physical therapy and the helpful nurses. He explained his philosophy that he had learned last year in hip surgery. I was blown away.

"It is important that right away you think straight, starting right after surgery. You have to program your mind to immediately be in the healing mode. If you wait too long the mind is already in the wrong direction and you feel worse. Keep your thinking straight from the get go. Don't let the negative get the tiniest grip."

Famous words, from my brother, Tom.

Millie on the other hand was the experimenter; always ready to try anything new and travel anyplace anytime. Tom preferred a quiet evening at home, while Millie preferred anything other than a quiet evening at home. It worked for them even though Millie complained most of the time. Tom planned to work until he was seventy-five and he couldn't understand why I had retired at fifty-five. He was my older brother. Millie, who was born in France, was a hard working homemaker. She had an easier time facing fantasy than reality. If she didn't like reality she made up fantasy and called it reality with a French twist. Their five children were each beautiful and kind souls. It had been a pleasure to watch them grow; two sons were in the armed services with one in Iraq; one daughter was married and teaching school, one a nurse and the youngest daughter in graduate school for psychology. All of the children lived in different states, the youngest attending school in California.

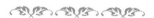

My grandparents and parents are deceased. My grandparents were farmers and had taught their eight children a strong work ethic. Both of my parents were the youngest in their families. I read the books on birth order and would be happy to state my beliefs about it. I believed it was a possible explanation for behavior, but not any more reliable than a flipped coin. I could continue on about free will and the importance of free will's role in life. I believed free will had consequences for each decision, which altered future decision-making. In other words the thoughts of today shaped the future and that was more powerful than birth order.

I had described my father as the typical old Irishman full of the dickens. As a youngster I never considered bringing a republican home to meet my father. My mother, on the other hand, was very German and could stretch a dollar better than any other living human being. My mother's childhood had not been easy in Germany. It was an extremely cold environment in many ways. My parents had learned to live with their differences probably for my brother and for my sake. I wouldn't say they were the happiest couple I ever knew. They loved us and I knew that for sure.

Chapter 5

Windows of the Mind

It was Sunday and another extremely beautiful day in Arizona. The temperature was in the mid-eighties and balmy. I wanted to be on the mountain hiking. I had called George to see if he could squeeze in a hike, but he was busy getting ready for his Thanksgiving trip to California. He was very close to his daughter and her family. I was glad George had lots of time now that he was retired to visit his family. I was going to miss him. George had some last words for me.

"Don't hike alone." It was a ritual for him to say this to me. I was a careful hiker; I have hiked alone within the city or on well-traveled trails. George knew I would hike alone but he said it anyway, it made him feel better or safer about me. We are sometimes like an old couple.

"I won't."

"Yes you will."

And, of course, I did.

This time of year was emotional for me. I did not have a lot of family in close proximity to Phoenix as they were scattered around the county. When I reached my regular hiking destination, I lifted the rear door of my Jeep Cherokee and changed into hiking boots. There weren't a lot of cars in the lot for such a beautiful day. I snapped my full fanny pack around my waist and crossed the street to the trailhead. Since it was Sunday I didn't expect to see anyone I knew. Regulars didn't hike on Sunday.

I felt an overwhelming sense of sadness as I climbed and couldn't quite put my finger on any cause. Things happened, I rationalized, that made me sad only to push me into change. Depression was a major symptom of the need for change. I trusted in my guiding spirit but depression was rearing its head. I complicated my life in so many ways. I didn't like the bureaucracy in any organizations or churches. Maybe I was anti-establishment. I told myself it was my personal ethics in conflict with group ethics. Neither was better than the other just different. In a church, I wondered who needed a bureaucracy to pray? The older I got, the less I believed that we needed someone else to tell us what to do or think. In the case of church and prayer it was God and the individual praying. I questioned if I carried dead weight on my shoulders by getting involved in the politics of any organization. I was sure that a lot of people in an organization could consider me dead weight.

I couldn't figure out why in past years I had been so judgmental of me. Then like a flash I remembered the darkest times in my life. As I navigated the depths of depression I always made myself wrong. Misfit meant something wrong with me. This awareness concretely confirmed my confidence in me. In past dark times I would hike as a way of processing and calming myself. There had been an association of hiking with depression. The association was negated. I hiked now in good times, my self-defined happy retirement. It interested me that twenty and thirty years ago I connected hiking with sadness. No wonder I took a thirty-year hiatus from hiking. As a retiree hiking was associated with fun and peace. Judgment is judgment. I prefer discernment. My goal was to observe what I felt. If I felt joy then I was on the right trail. If there were two mountains joy and sadness then I would choose joy. No way would I spend time hiking sadness. The same went for two mountains named scared and sacred. It was a waste of my time to beat myself up.

In the next breath my new prayer sewed a new seed for new growth. I decided on a seed of focus in the present moment. Let the past be the past and the future the future. Right here right now. The energy had shifted and my depression was gone. While the amount of change is constructive, the direction of change is the most important. Awareness changed things in a positive direction.

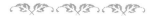

Back in late spring I went to a spiritual psychic who told me I would move in August. The psychic saw me packing boxes and ready to journey. Through the years my working summers had become longer and hotter. I was definitely ready for change and it wasn't a bad idea to move away from the heat of Phoenix. It could have been the power of suggestion more than a psychic read.

I made a mental list of possible places to move. There was Kentucky, Ohio, California, New Mexico, Alaska, and northern Arizona. My parameters were flimsy; I like the southwest, and places where family or friends live. Another possibility was Switzerland where Jessica lived. We were best friends through elementary school, high school, and college. She was an environmental engineer stationed in Zurich and worked for a private corporation. I had visited her on several occasions and we both had taken a cruise in Alaska. Jessica was my oldest friend in the world. She lived in a three bedroom, two bathroom flat with her husband and dog. They were family to me.

Along with the move the idea of potential identity came to my mind. New place, new identity, new life; retirement creates all types of choices. It wouldn't be too complicated to change my identity especially if I moved. That could be fun and interesting. I chuckled and laughed out loud. Changing my identity was sneaky and interesting at the same time. I considered myself a gentle person with nothing to hide. The adventure of it attracted me. It wasn't much of a stretch to imagine it but doing it lacked purpose. I had to think about that and my definition of fun.

I wasn't sure what, if anything, I was looking for in an identity change. Years ago in a workshop I surmised that I always searched and searched for what I believed I didn't have. In reality I was looking for me the way I was before I had learned to pretend to be what I wasn't. It sounded like how I feel about the mountain people.

Chapter 6

A New Identity

I watched a movie many years ago about a female psychiatrist who experimented with her alter ego. In the daytime she dressed conservatively for work and at night she went out dressed like a cheap floozy. She conducted the experiment under the guise of clinical research on herself. She became so mesmerized by her alter ego that she got herself into deep trouble and was eventually murdered. That was a hypothesis to think about. The alter ego could be a preferred place to live from rather than from the ego self. It could be dangerous playing around with a fantasy of changed identity. Right now I preferred being the who "me" really was. And I was curious about other facets of me.

It was funny that I could literally disappear and no one would know for some time. Nancy, in a double life, could go on for many years without detection. I've read about men being married to multiple wives who knew nothing of the existence of the other wives. I have never read about women who have done the same thing, but it was possible. The irony of a single, never married woman marrying simultaneous husbands was not lost but, not fun. A changed identity could be revealing like an espionage event of the self on the self. I could rationalize anything.

I could see me signing up for a new social security card, and bank account. My pension check would remain in my name unless I did a formal name change, but then what the heck? My true thought was that only criminals and tired spouses changed their identity.

My mind swirled with silly ideas; such as maybe I was avoiding something else? Maybe I would have a related dream tonight. Driving to the store I became aware of all the different types of vehicles on the freeway. If I changed identity then I would need new wheels. I could become a conservative or a liberal. Maybe the easiest thing was to buy a motor home and take off. I could keep my own identify but have a road name; like a CB radio name or handle. I called my friends who owned a motor home and began questioning. It was a short conversation as they were camping in Prescott. There are motor homes with motors like class A, B, C, and travel trailers that might hitch to the back of a truck. Travel trailers do not have motors. A new identity on wheels; this could be fun. It seemed like too much work not to be honest. I would have to remember a bunch of stretched truths or lies.

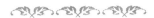

That night I dreamt about airplanes and helicopters that kept flying around a mountain diving and rising up over the setting sun. The only other thing I remembered about the dream was this big beautiful mountain. It didn't mean too much to me at the time but I tape-recorded my memories of it anyway.

Chapter 7

Morning Coffee

Morning coffee in my yard under the old mesquite tree is always an alternative to a hike. My motor home loving neighbors, peddled by on their bikes. Some mornings they stopped and other mornings they yelled hello and continued on with their ride. I hadn't talked to them since they returned from Prescott.

"Hey good morning."

Frieda steered her bike into my driveway. Ben was right behind her and gave a wave. Ben was a man of few words and very quick wit. He was one of the salt of the earth guys. Frieda was earthy and all the good things a person could be. She was as real as they come; a get what you see type of gal and proud of it. They belonged to an international camping group that gathered about eight times a year for four or five days in the southwest. Activities included potlucks, hiking, touring and many games. We have been friends for ten years and they are extended family to me.

"Wait till you hear what we did, we hiked and played all kinds of board games. And next time Nancy we want you to come with us."

I chuckled and reminded them that I snored loudly and made frequent trips to the bathroom.

Frieda laughed. "We could run into each other en route".

I told them about the gal down the street who had sold her house for big bucks and bought a condo in Tucson.

"She bought a condo in Tucson and now wants a Winnebago to drive to Montana. She wants to be back for her mother's nine-tieth birthday."

Ben caught my eye. "When are you going to do the same thing?"

"Me, no way, I like a real bathroom. When you ride your bike by the neighbor's house you will see her; she is busy organizing, packing, and getting ready to leave."

In my mind I had decided it wouldn't be difficult for me to plan a fantasy trip in a motor home. I must have laughed out loud because Frieda questioned me.

"What's so funny?"

"Just life."

Frieda and Ben left on their bikes. "Think about going with us next time Nancy."

"Yeah yeah."

Life was a mystery and the more freedom I had, the more confusion it created, or so it seemed to me. I remembered a "What the Bleep" study group at a Unity Church in Paradise Valley that I had attended a couple of years ago. I had heard the phrase "realm of potential" likened to hundreds of basketballs bouncing all at the same time and a person choosing the one he wanted. That was potential. If I turned my head and focused on one of the basketball potentials that potential would change to experience. That one ball would shift from potential to my experience. Only one at a time of the potentials could become experience. The rest remained in potential status ready to spring. Focusing on one thought caused the shift. If that were so then my potential place to live right now was geographically everywhere. My experience would begin when I concentrated on one potential, moving it from potential to experience. This was what I concluded from what I had heard. It worked for me. I would swim in potential for a while and see what popped up for me. I thought the same for my name, and my identity. Potentially many names, old and new, existed. Life was a trip and for the first time in a long time I felt I had the freedom to take off into as many directions as I could choose.

In many of the philosophical books that I have read the authors investigated the physical and the dream worlds. Many thought the dream world was more real than the physical world. "Life is but a dream" was an old phrase. I knew that dreams were significant in my life. The dream world was very creative. Maybe my dreams tonight would provide more explanation on the airplanes and helicopters dream from the previous night.

Chapter 8

The Mountain Speaks

Monday morning I was on my way to climb the mountain again. As I drove I decided that my climb would be happy. Last time I climbed I had fallen into some old negative stuff. It was good that I healed it, but I wanted today to be a light and happy hike. I decided in that moment that I was choosing happy thoughts. An affirmation I used earlier in the month was "I am loving who I am and choosing to be here fully." At least that was the best I could recall it without going home to look up what I had written. That meant I didn't affirm it too many times or it would have been committed to memory. It was time for affirmation now.

On the mountain I decided to change my climbing pattern and hiked up the back way, opposite direction from the old riding stables. I reminded myself about my goal of happy thoughts. My subconscious kicked in after a short time and before I knew it my thoughts were negative. It didn't take long. At that exact second I tripped on a rock and almost fell. My trip brought me back to the present moment. I tripped physically just as I had tripped into a negative thought. I thought it was pretty bizarre. It happened again under the same circumstances. I drifted off into negative land and this time my hand braced my fall. Thank God it was uphill and not downhill. It was harder to catch myself falling downhill. My subconscious and the mountain brought me back on the trail into the now moment. Back on the trail or path what a lovely thought. Life was a path.

I remembered a dream George had shared with me when he first retired.

George, in a slick gold and white tuxedo, had four groomsmen dressed in lavender suits. They were all climbing to the top of a mountain. It was a very hot day and there was no path or trail to follow just rocks. They were trailblazing in their finest clothes. When they reached the top there was a resort and as George looked down at the Valley from the top of the mountain he saw a road that came up the mountain and he became irritated at himself in the dream because he could have driven up the mountain instead of hiking up it in his wedding tux.

Mountains seemed to reveal much, in so many ways. If one followed how water flowed down a mountain one could see the best way to etch a path for going up the mountain. It probably was how the path I was hiking evolved. I heard that in Oak Creek Canyon the ranchers followed how cattle descended. Cattle always figured out the easiest way to forge a trail. I laughed because the cattle poop allowed a human nose to follow their trail. In the past when I hiked Grand Canyon the stench of Donkey poop on the path was a daily experience. It reassured me that I was on the right path. Back to George's dream; at the end of my own life I might look back over my life path and realize there had been an easier way. In his dream they got up the mountain the best way they knew. Once up there it was easier to see from a bird's eye view a better way. The party on top was the same whatever way they came up. They wore wedding clothes for a reason, some celebration. If I knew then what I knew now then I would have done better; or at least taken the easier path. They got where they wanted to go. Life was grand.

Up ahead on the trail was Ted and he was waving and waited for me to catch up. He looked anxious to tell me something and I guessed it was about his new grandchild. I was glad to see him so happy.

"Hey Ted, how is it going?"

"Better, we are going the same direction and I have good news."

Today was a day for a happy climb without tripping into negativity. Ted broke my spell with his comment.

"Think we woke the snakes up?"

I loved all this free time that allowed the serendipity of the moment to unfold. My mind could shift so easily from positive to negative.

Chapter 9

Motor Homes

The freedom to become someone other than myself continued to intrigue me. Originally it had shocked me. I truly loved who I was but there was mystery as to what lived on the other side of the known, like the other side of a mountain. It was the old "grass is greener on the other side." Something was sexy about freedom to change to transform into someone else. It was risky and strange because that someone could be unlikable.

Thoughts of cruising around in a motor home occupied me and I decided to call Frieda again.

"Hi Frieda listen what types of motor home do you think I could handle for short trips around the state?"

"A Kodiak."

It was a van vehicle with one room and a mini bathroom. One didn't have to leave the vehicle to start it up. You could get out of bed and jump in the driver seat and take off. As a solo female it was important to me in case I needed a quick get away. If I needed to go outside to get in the drivers seat it would be self defeating. I didn't want any helpless feelings. In reality if someone was after me it I guessed it wouldn't make much difference, they could slash tires or whatever. I questioned myself ad nausea about silly things like where I would park a vehicle. Parking my vehicle in the middle of a forest was highly unlikely.

What I really wanted in a vehicle would cost a half million dollars. The likelihood of me driving any type of motor home, class C or Kodiak was minimal. I don't like to drive. When the weather is hot and stuffy I get sleepy to the sound of a constant motor. One time driving from Monterey, California to Phoenix, I drove eighteen hours straight and ingested diet coke by the gallon to keep awake. I needed to rethink my identity change. It wasn't sounding fun any longer.

Some people connect motor homes with trailer trash. As a child I may have thought that way, but no more. For one thing these vehicles were very expensive and one needed a lot of money to make a purchase. Knowing people like Frieda and Ben demonstrated the goodness of people who chose this lifestyle.

One very old belief system related to motor homes popped up for me. It was long forgotten. My memory flashed back to the early seventies when a friend of a friend from out of state visited me. The friend asked to park his small motor home in front of my apartment. Since my apartment was in the back of the complex his parking by my front door conveniently hid his motor home. I hesitated before saying yes because I knew the landlord did not approve of motor homes on the premises. He parked in front of my door and I showed him around my complex. Who knows why, but I pointed out the scary hidden locations where robbers could break into other people's apartments and no one would see the break in. I thought it was strange that he took such an interest in that subject. The friend of a friend was gone the next morning along with his motor home presumably packed with items he had stolen from my neighbors. The police were at my door the next day asking if I saw anything unusual since so many places had been broken into the night before in my area. I gave the police the little information I had about him. That was my personal connection to motor homes. Needless to say I quickly revised that old belief system. Although I did wonder whatever happened to the friend of a friend or if the police even found him.

I cannot place myself in a new identity or a fantasy that included a motor home. It was not realistic. Again it crossed my mind that opening the door to fantasy could be dangerous. Steven King novels were superb in this venue. Imagination came from deep within. Even Einstein talked about imagination and its power. Imagination was not something I could physically put in my hand but I knew it existed. And I knew I was free to explore it all.

Show Low, Arizona was an interesting name for a town and it made me smile when I spoke it. Show Low got its name from a poker game and, just like it sounded, showed low. Maybe somewhere else there were towns named straight or royal flush. I looked up the town Show Low on the Internet. The temperature appeared to be similar to Flagstaff, which meant snow in the winter. It might be cool to spend a summer there I thought. Maybe my plan to change identity would come to fruition there. My devil's advocate interjected I didn't know anyone there so a changed identity would have no purpose. Because I can, was my thought. It was a silly rationale. Maybe I could rent an apartment under an assumed name. It would be easier to go under my own name and be a different Nancy. My ideas got sillier. I was deeply appreciative of being free to have the idea. In any event I could plan a long weekend trip and check out the local real estate in Show Low. Freedom always had an answer. It is a mountain with lots of trails.

Chapter 10

Granola and Brownies

It was Wednesday and I was back on my healing mountain. Everyone paused along the trail to talk about the upcoming Thursday interview with the reporter.

"Hey Nancy, did you hear what is going on tomorrow?"

Five times I was asked that question. All the regular hikers and many of the occasional hikers had wind of the interview and that a newspaper reporter was doing a story on the mountain. The mountain was buzzing. Ted, Stan, Sue, Ginny, and the other hikers that I don't even know by name convinced me to show up

"At least come for the picture taking at the top of the mountain, you don't have to talk."

Some of the hikers planned to bring treats like granola bars. I smiled in amazement

"Hikers are so hip you guys think of everything natural, even granola bars".

Some mentioned bringing their dogs. This was turning into a party. Some hikers I saw on the trail I didn't recognize, but what the heck, it would be fun with new people. Maybe they normally hiked later in the day. It would be great to be with the regulars all at one time in one place. I turned to Ted.

"Oh yeah, where is Jareed and his sidekick dog, Shade? Surely he heard about the interview."

"You know, Nance, Jareed is Muslim. He may not be comfortable with the attention or a picture in a newspaper. A lot of people have their private stories and we may never know their histories."

I nodded to Ted. "Ever been to Show Low?"

"Show Low! That's where my granddaughter is moving to after their honeymoon. How is that for a small world and why do you ask?"

Ted had a great smile that lit up his rugged face. His sky blue eyes, visible now that he wasn't wearing sunglasses, glistened in the sun. Ted liked the small town atmosphere in Show Low. In past conversations with him I knew he and his wife had traveled the world. He was a computer whiz and had worked in Saudi, Arabia for twenty-three years. Living in Arabia conditioned and prepared him to be able to hike in the summer desert of Arizona when the temperature was a hundred twenty degrees.

Ted would have been a great spy; he had that swagger of intelligence and a sharp wit. He could easily have been involved in espionage. Espionage would be more intriguing than computers. He would never voluntarily tell me if he was in espionage because it wasn't any of my business. My attention returned to hiking in the present moment on my healing mountain. A family of quail crossed in front of us. Ted was first to become aware of our bird visitors.

"Excuse us little quail for getting in your way."

He pointed to the quail. The quail ignored us. We both laughed. Ted and I laughed a lot on hikes. I enjoyed his company. Too bad he was married; on second thought if he was single we would still be friends. Friends were great!! We finished the hike and planned to meet tomorrow to hike together for the big gathering on top of the mountain with the reporter.

"Get here early Nancy, if you want a parking place?"

"Yeah, I wouldn't want to miss the picture taking."

"I hear sarcasm."

"See you tomorrow." We hugged as we parted.

When I got home I played my phone messages. Frieda had left a message about a great deal on a small used motor home.

"It is a steal and the perfect size for you to drive" was the message. It wouldn't hurt me just to look at it. I pushed the button to call the sender on the phone and picked up a pad of paper for writing information. Frieda had caller id and answered.

"Ben and I will drive you to the lot. He is interested in looking at another motor home at the same place."

"Great."

They both were experts on motor homes and I appreciated their assistance. After I hung up I began thinking about my finances and questioned my ability to afford one. I needed to know what I could realistically purchase. When I was indecisive I longed for a partner to help with the decision-making. Sometimes I got tired of doing all the ordinary stuff myself like getting gas, washing the car, and paying the bills. On second thought if I had a partner I couldn't play with the thought of changing my identity. Immediately I was glad I was who I was.

Later that evening at the Copper Star Coffee Shop I met friends from a woman's writing retreat. Together we represented married, single, divorced, gay or lesbian, straight, and young to old: me the oldest. Our common thread was writing and any theme evoked discussion. One lady, Steph, treasured always being devil's advocate. This night the subject of intimacy came up. We ordered our coffee, dessert and waited by the counter for our orders. One by one we sat in squeaky cushiony seats and rolled up under a round table careful not to spill or drop a morsel. The sounds of clanging dishes and chatter were all around us. The room noises faded when our subject deepened and interest was keen. We didn't hear anyone else but I am sure they heard us. My nose could almost smell cigarette or cigar smoke through the heavy coffee aromas but smoking wasn't allowed in Arizona restaurants. When I smoked this was the time I lit up. Thank God I gave that up. We called ourselves the five Ss and an N; Sally, Sara, Sue, Steph, Serena, and Nancy. Sally was the conservative of the group, a staunch republican, married for twenty-five years and a mother of two. Sara had been through a bad divorce last year at age thirty. Sue was forty something, gay, and in a committed partnership for five years. Steph, with her spiked red hair, was harder to describe; at twenty-two years of age she didn't fit into any of the groups I was familiar with. She experienced the spectrum of sexuality or so she said. Serena, in a new relationship, was a thirty-two year old single mom of a thirteen-year-old boy. And I, Nancy, was the retiree of the group. Everyone else worked. We could discuss pencils and it would get exciting. We tossed around politics and moved to intimacy.

Steph forked into her double chocolate brownie. "If words create things why can't I create more intimacy with the lovers in my life? Everyone is so afraid of mistakes or they run scared when the subject comes up."

Serena sipped her mocha. "You could and would if you really wanted it in your life. You camouflage your fear of intimacy by surrounding yourself with so many and then blame them. Intimacy takes time. Ted and I have been dating for a year now. It is scary to be open and honest. Lots of times I'm thinking about what he wants me to say rather than what is true for me. I can't imagine trying to be open with more than one lover at a time."

Steph rolled her eyes. "You guys live in the dark ages. There is a whole spectrum of sexuality out there."

Sally stirred her tea. "You are going back to the dark ages where people lived in caves like animals and did whatever, whenever. I just read a book on intention; Steph, do you think you could set an intention for yourself and be open to experiencing intimacy with one partner? I've been married to the same man for many years; there is no way I could create what I have with him if there were more than one man in my life." Steph was cool.

"Sally, you may want to experiment being with more than one. I'm kidding and I'm listening to you guys, I may not agree but I'm listening."

Sara offered to share her cookies. "It is easier for me to date several men rather than just one. It is like all my eggs are in one basket. But Sally is right, I loose the sense of intimacy by dating several, but there is less probability I will be hurt. I don't put myself out there in intimacy. My divorce was painful and I don't want to go there again."

Sue smiled. "No one likes to be hurt. Imagine how I as a gay person feel about not being able to legally marry. I went through the whole dating thing; found intimacy and can't marry because of my sexuality. That hurts." She shifted her gaze to Sally. "And don't even go to the procreation theory Sally, lots of straight people marry as older adults, they can't pro-create either. You all heard about what is happening in California where the gay couples are refusing to pay taxes if they can't legally marry."

Sally was eagerly waiting to break in.

"Hold on Sue, I am in favor of recognizing partner rights just not marriage." Steph didn't miss a beat.

"You two need to have intimate understanding and acceptance of each other except I agree with Sue. You know Sally; no one tells you, you can't marry. Don't even tell me that every time you made love you had the intention of having children. You probably can't reproduce anymore and I bet you are still making love? The word lovemaking sounds weird but if I use the "f" word you all will really freak out. So Nancy, you are the oldest one here what do you think?"

"I never got the intimacy thing down pat, but I am still working on it."

Steph and Sue howled; the others just smiled, like Cheshire cats.

"The whole concept of intimacy is evolving in the older single population. Love the second or third time around is pretty focused. Others, like me, are retired and have lots of time and energy to do and to travel. There is a well founded fear of sexually transmitted diseases in the older population." Sara was wise.

"So Nancy what is it you want that you don't have?"

"Get to the point will you, Sara? Up until now my problem has been I didn't know myself well enough. How can someone get to know me when I don't know and love myself? I had to learn I wasn't perfect. My refuge was work. Now I am into fun and exploring. Like Steph, I want to create intimacy with everyone. It isn't sex although sex is part of it. With sex I am still one on one. When you sleep with someone you sleep with every other person they have slept with. Talk about risk." Steph always said whatever came to her mind.

"Let's talk about masturbation." As a joke Sally stood up to leave but Serena persisted.

"That's self-pleasure and not a relationship, get a toy, I like discussing intimacy." Sally smiled.

"I am so glad we can agree to disagree. This group stimulates me. I appreciate so much that you respect my opinions especially you, Sue. I don't approve of gay marriage and you don't condemn me. You are right I don't understand gay people. I am working on it and knowing you is helping me"

I looked around the table at my good friends and took a moment to be grateful for good conversation.

"To answer what is missing, nothing is missing in my life. Most days on a scale from one to ten I run around nine. It would enhance my life to share with another and lead me to the realm of eleven. Of course meditation does that some days. The simple act of holding hands or knowing each other's thoughts is gratifying. I listen to what Sally says about her husband of twenty-five years. It couldn't have been easy, but through the years they know each other. Just like Sue and Gail, they know each other to a much deeper degree after five years. Time can do a lot of things. My journey is mine and I wouldn't trade it."

The owner, Bill, was closing up and gave us a ten-minute till closing signal. Sue offered a suggestion. "Before we meet again let's each set and write an intention about intimacy in our life, we could set it and write about the evolvement and unfolding of it. What do you think?"

Everyone nodded except Sally.

"I like it and I think I will focus my intimacy intention on my relationship with my children." Sue's eyes lit up.

"You know Sally, you could create intimacy with me and learn more about the gay population and I could learn more about you. Give it some thought. Hey we could write a book together. When shall we all meet again, want to do next month same time and place?"

We all agreed.

Chapter 11

Press Conference on the Mountain

Thursday was here and I drove to the mountain. I missed George and wished he were still in town. He would have climbed with us if he were here, but he was having a ball with his grandchildren. I made a mental note to cut out the article whenever it appeared in the newspaper to give to George when he returned. I would make several copies to give or send to interested family and friends. I talked a lot to many people about my healing mountain. I truly believed the mountain had healing powers.

Laughter bubbled up in my psyche because here I was making fantasy plans about changing my identity and at the same time was planning to cut out articles with possible pictures and comments from me on my healing mountain. This was something to rationalize and pretty silly. Yes, I was free to be silly. "Life was grand" was my theme in retirement. I pulled into the crowded parking lot. The first person I saw was Jareed with his dog Shade. Jareed and Shade had crossed the street and were at the trailhead. There were a few other people standing in the lot; I didn't know them and had never seen them before. I maneuvered my jeep into a parking space. I looked around but didn't see any sign of the reporter or any semblance of a photographer. I was a little late and, maybe, they all had headed up. I decided to head on up the mountain knowing I was late. The party would be in progress when I reached the top. My planned party time at the top was half an hour max. My intention was to hike. I was there to hike. As usual I mapped out in my mind, which way I would go up and come down.

The day was beautiful with sunshine and a pleasant breeze. It was quietly majestic. Everyone I passed or who passed me on the trail was unusually friendly. This was different. I realized many times hikers are deep in their own thoughts and hardly noticed another hiker on the trail. After about forty minutes I reached the top and, wow, nearly all the comfortable rocks to sit on were taken. That was an oxymoron, rocks and comfortable seats. I looked around and saw familiar faces, Stan, Jareed, Sue, Abe, Tina but no Ted. We all waved to one another. An additional ten or so people were there most of whom I had seen on the trail. My eyes landed on the granola bars and I reached for one.

"Thank you whoever brought these." There were lots of extra water bottles but no reporter.

"Is George coming?" Stan came over to join me and share my granola bar.

"No, he's on vacation visiting his grandchildren in California."

"Is he visiting his son-in-law, the one in the marines"?

I nodded my head as I crunched on the granola bar. George was so proud of his son-in-law. He even pasted a marine sticker on the bumper of his car.

As we spoke I saw the reporter drag himself around a corner, but no photographer was with him, at least not yet.

He gave a wave to the group. He looked tired, winded and thirsty. Sue handed him a bottle of water and fluffed her hair.

"Where's the photographer? I fixed my hair special."

We all laughed. The reporter held up a digital camera, actually, a Nikon like mine. I knew it was a good camera and probably on loan to him from the newspaper. The reporter sat down.

"I need a few minutes to rest, anyone object?"

Stan spoke for the group. "Of course not. You out of shape?"

The reporter ignored us and kept looking out over the valley. We circled around him. He drank his water and spoke with us.

"This is a bird's eye view. It is beautiful up here. I can see why you all climb here every day."

I observed the reporter who was in awe of the view. He seemed to have put the labor of the trek up the mountain in his past. He pulled out his notes from last week and began reviewing who had said what.

"I'm verifying names and quotes because I want to quote you folks correctly."

He wrote down our full names with phone numbers so he could contact us later if necessary. He took pictures and we smiled until our teeth hurt. Even the dogs were in the pictures. It would be hard to pick me out in any picture as I wore a wide brimmed hat. The shade from the hat alone hid my face. The reporter looked up amid his pile of paperwork.

"Where's Ted?" I looked around as if to confirm Ted's absence.

"Ted was planning on being here, something must have come up. He is either late or you may even see him on your way down the mountain."

The reporter thanked us all for the story.

"If you don't mind I'm going to sit here for awhile and enjoy the view. It beats the view of my messy desk."

I hung around a little while, maybe five minutes. Five minutes was enough time to let the faster hikers go ahead. I was pretty slow on the way down. It was easier to let people go ahead of me in mass than it was to keep pulling over on the side to let them pass. I had hiking this mountain down to an art.

In my five minutes of waiting to descend I watched the reporter and all he did was write on his pad. He wasn't even looking at the view as he had said he wanted to do. Maybe that was how he got us to shut up so he could finish his report. I wondered why he hadn't just brought a computer up here; that would have been easier and natural for a reporter. I tried to figure out why he didn't enjoy the place for a while, but he didn't, at least not in my five minutes of observation. It was none of my business and I headed on down my healing mountain. I could have brought my camera to take a picture of the reporter to show my interested friends. It would have been a picture of a story in the making. I loved this mountain. It is always different yet always the same wisdom every time I have climbed it. I decided to enjoy the view.

A man with a big hat approached me and I thought it might be Ted but it wasn't. I hoped Ted connected with the reporter. Ted was very intelligent and an all around good guy. When I reached the parking lot I looked for Ted's car. It wasn't there. Something must have come up. Next time I saw Ted, he would tell me all about it.

I stopped at the grocery store on the way home and picked up some stuff to make bean tacos. Tacos were definitely southwest. I remembered the first time I ate a taco back when I was twenty years old on vacation in California. I incorrectly pronounced the words taco and guacamole. I thought refried beans looked like something someone had already eaten. Twenty years later I loved refried beans. If I took on a new identity I could be from back east and have never heard about Mexican food. If only I could speak Spanish; that would be cool. I knew a little and actually had some Spanish in high school, but I knew my talents were not in learning languages. It might be a good time to change an old belief system and learn a new language.

I arrived home and my message light was flashing. I listened while I put away the groceries. It was Frieda.

"How is the search for a motor home coming along? Good deals go fast, if you truly are interested Nancy, you need to make a move. Call the owner and at least go look at it."

I reached for my phone.

"Thank you Frieda, I'm going to call the seller after I hang up from leaving this message, but I don't know how committed I am to making a purchase. Look for the newspaper article about the mountain."

Last year Frieda and Ben climbed the mountain with me. It wasn't something they particularly liked to do but they loved traveling in motor homes. I was glad to have such mobile friends. After I hung up I looked at the newspaper ad for the motor home. I dialed the number. This was going to be very interesting.

Chapter 12

Back to the Club

Everyone has kick back and do nothing days. I had a lot of them now that I was in the ranks of the retired. I decided to go to the Club and the whole gang was there. A regular group works out on Monday, Wednesday and Friday mornings. Gina and Charles are the volunteer social directors. It was a few days before Thanksgiving and Gina was already talking about who was bringing what to our neighborhood feast. This year we would gather at my house in the side yard. It was a perfect place for outdoor eating as there was a one hundred year old mesquite tree grove that shaded a couple of old iron tables. The shading was perfect. History had it that the area was an old Hohokum Indian dwelling. Supposedly the area by my house was their garbage dump. I was sure it held treasure and I was always going to put a metal detector to the test. Next year I kept telling myself, next year. Anyway Gina invited the Club to our potluck. Fortunately everyone had plans. That many people would not fit comfortably in my yard. Everyone at the Club was in a good mood. I had a great workout, which meant an hour on machines and an hour on the treadmill.

After the Club I went to the store and returned home. I pulled into my driveway and noticed Larry, my neighbor, walking his dog, Nut. This was the first time in several weeks that I had the opportunity to speak with Larry. I got out of the car.

"Hi Larry, how are you doing?"

We hadn't chatted for a while so we talked for a half an hour about local gossip and the weather. Larry did some sharing on a personal note.

"I didn't sleep last night because my wife was up half the night."

Larry and Beth had been married for sixty-nine years. Sixty-nine years were longer than I had been on the earth. I hadn't even celebrated a one-year anniversary let alone sixty-nine. Larry and his wife had spent every summer for the past thirty years in Strawberry, Arizona. Strawberry was a very small town northeast of Phoenix.

"Is everything okay?"

"You know Nancy, last year Beth and I came back from Strawberry earlier than we wanted or planned. Beth was ill; she had that pain from Shingles and we thought she was going to have to be hospitalized. Fortunately it didn't go that way, but she is pretty sick. She sleeps all the time and she has no energy."

Larry looked a little pale. I was concerned.

"How are you handling all this? What does your doctor say?"

"Right now I am more concerned about Beth. These doctors don't know what to say, they just give you lots of medicine."

I pressed him for more information. "What about you Larry, how are you?"

"Very tired, I keep thinking about the cabin and all the fun we have had there. Our lives are changing; at least Beth's is changing. I don't think she is capable of going up north and I can't leave her. It is shattering. Strawberry is such a part of our lives."

Larry paused and just looked off into the sky. "I don't care about going to the cabin ever without Beth. She is sick this year. I would like to just get up there to clean it. We left it in shambles, we were in a hurry to leave, and it's a mess. And Nancy it is all replaceable."

What an attitude he had. He remained positive even though his wife was quite ill. Material things mean less and less to me as I age. When someone you love is ill those things mean nothing unless you had to sell them to pay bills. The concern on his face made me want to cry.

"If I can help let me know, I could stay with Beth or drive up with you."

"Our neighbors there in Strawberry offered to do whatever we needed last year. I just shut and locked the door and prayed."

"Maybe you could give them a call."

Larry gave a small chuckle. His face was worried.

"Now in November most all the neighbors have returned to the valley for winter, most of them were there just for summer. They get out of the heat. Some live in Tucson, some in Mesa, or Chandler, you know the general Phoenix area. Up there everyone is within three miles of one another. Here in the valley some are a couple of hours drive."

"Hey, I'd be happy to drive to Strawberry to check things out for you if you like? It would be great for me to get away up north. I don't think I've ever been to Strawberry."

Larry got a big grin on his face.

"That's a possibility and I just may take you up on it."

Larry and Beth had been my neighbors for twenty some years, which is about as long as they had gone to Strawberry for summers. I had celebrated their fiftieth and sixtieth anniversaries. They had supported me through my losses. I was there for them when they lost the oldest of their three daughters in a car accident. The middle daughter and son-in-law lived oversees, the youngest daughter and son-in-law lived in New Mexico. Their children, grandchildren and great grandchildren all lived out of state. Larry and Beth had four great-grand children. They were family to me. I was the next-door neighbor and it was easy and convenient for me to fill in for the out of town kids.

I invited Larry and Beth for Thanksgiving. With Beth being sick I knew they wouldn't be going to their daughter's in New Mexico, which they normally did for Thanksgiving. I thought the two of them might enjoy spending time with us, their neighbors. Our neighborhood is very comfortable, no driving necessary, and we weren't too noisy.

"I'll check with Beth and let you know about Thanksgiving."

We parted ways and I headed into the house. I tried to catch the phone but I missed it.

"Oh well".

On my machine was a message from the couple selling the motor home. The owners offered me an appointment for ten on Friday morning. Of course they wanted me to bring Ben and Frieda along to see the rig. I had learned so much about the language of motor homes. Motor homes were big and something I truly did not want to drive but I was fascinated. In my pre-retirement condition I would never have spent time researching something I didn't think would happen. In retirement I could go down any road I wanted to and learn about all kinds of things.

Travel trailers folded up and could be hauled by a truck or a jeep. When a person reached his destination it could be detached, raised up and extended out, and ready to go. It could transform from a squashed pancake to a large trailer. I thought it was magic and thought I could do that if I wanted.

I called the lady selling the travel trailer and confirmed the appointment. Next I called Frieda and Ben to check their availability. Frieda was quick to respond to my request.

"Sure no problem, we'll go with you. Guess what Ben and I are doing?"

"Are you buying another trailer?"

"No we're putting a concrete slab in the backyard so we have room to park the motor home and the travel trailer. We aren't comfortable with the motor home or the TravelManor parked in the driveway."

Her comment made me think about where I would park anything I might purchase. Their yard had a cement wall around the backyard and a wonderful watchdog, Angel. I had no fence and no dog. I did have a cat named Tweetie. Tweetie slept most of the day and most of the night for that matter. Buying a travel trailer was becoming a pipe dream.

Chapter 13

Thanksgiving Time

The next few days were pretty standard for me. I did my routine at the Club and climbed the mountain. On one of my climbs Ted and I hiked the whole way around the mountain twice as we had several times the year before. We shared our personal ups and downs in life. The mountain was a safe place to become vulnerable and we opened up.

"Ted, where were you? You missed the reporter you know."

"It sounds like an excuse, but we got unexpected company from out of town."

"I don't buy it Ted; it isn't like you needed to be with that company all day."

He ignored me and I let it go.

"So where is the article Nancy? I keep looking for it in the newspaper. Did you scare him away?"

"Very funny Ted." It was always fun to be around Ted, he kept a light heart.

"I haven't seen it yet either. I keep looking for it. With everything else going on in Phoenix I wouldn't be surprised if the article is on a back burner."

Ted was very conservative and a believer in the war in Iraq. I was a liberal. We respected and trusted each other even though we were opposites. Discussing the war in Iraq was off limits. We wished each other Happy Thanksgiving. I looked forward to talking with Ted more after the holiday.

"Nancy, if you get to Show Low promise you will look up my granddaughter? Here I'll write down the number for you."

I had met his grand daughter once when she had hiked with us.

"Thanks Ted, I just may do that."

Pretty cool I thought, especially if I get to go to Strawberry. I would have to look up the distance from Strawberry to Show Low. I never did hear back from Larry about going to clean up his cabin for him.

Thanksgiving was very laid back, plenty of great food and pleasant neighbors. Neighbors walked by and stopped to say hello. There were six of us for dinner and about twelve more for dessert. Thanksgiving was calm and peaceful in other words it was uneventful.

Chapter 14

The Day after Thanksgiving

I heard an ambulance and it was no surprise that it pulled up next door to Larry and Beth's house. No one else in the neighborhood appeared to be surprised, but we were all concerned for Beth's health.

That evening, after he returned from the hospital, Larry stopped briefly in my yard and gave me a report on Beth.

"Beth is going to be in the Intensive Care Unit for awhile".

"Is there anything any of us can do to help you?"

"No, not with Beth, God and the doctors are doing that." He paused and looked me straight in the eyes. "Were you serious about driving to Strawberry to check on the cabin for me? The grandkids all live out of town and I can't leave Beth."

"Sure Larry, it would be fun for me. Tell you what; I could go up in couple of days if you like. How about I come over at your convenience and you tell me exactly what you want checked on at the cabin? It would give you some time to think about what you want me to do."

I saw relief on Larry's face. He didn't ask for help often and it warmed my heart to be of comfort to him. Something fun for me, like go to Strawberry, helped him out. It was a win win situation. Inside my heart I committed to be there for him. He was my friend.

"It would mean a lot to me, there are some private things I want out of the cabin. I'll get a list together. Right now I need some sleep, Beth is doing well and the doctors sent me home."

The next morning Larry called me.

"Can you come over around seven tonight? I'll have a map and some other things for you along with the keys of course. It will be cold up there you know, are you sure you don't mind?"

"Honest Larry, it's fine, I need an adventure. I'll see you at seven tonight."

It was a beautiful breezy evening in Phoenix and I made my way over to Larry's. I rang the doorbell and patiently waited for a sound or some indication that Larry had heard. "Larry?" I called out and a few seconds later I heard the familiar sound of the latch unlocking and Nut barking.

"Hi Nancy, come on in."

I handed Larry a package wrapped in aluminum foil.

"I made some pumpkin bread for you. It's warm, fresh from the oven. How is Beth doing today?"

Larry took the bread.

"Thank you. That air feels crisp out there." He closed the door. "Look we both have sweaters on. Beth is doing quite well, and may be moved out of ICU."

"I'm so glad; you know your neighbors are here for you. Maybe we could help with meals or shopping especially when she comes home."

"You remember Lucy? She's the gal who cleans for us. I called her and she can come twice a week if we need it. She has a key to the house too. I think I have it covered." He pointed to the dining room table and invited me to sit. I could see papers stacked neatly in piles. I sat and he began.

"Here is the map to the cabin and the keys. These two keys are the same, either one will open both the front and the side door. I don't know why I keep them together but I do. This third odd shaped key I will explain as I go along. Now behind the cabin are the propane tanks, the septic tanks and whatever other kind of tanks there might be."

We both laughed.

"Are there any nearby motels? I prefer not dealing with any tanks? I assume I'd have to if I stayed in the cabin."

"The cabin has a fireplace which could keep you plenty warm."

"I love fireplaces, enjoying a fire in a fireplace balances out fiddling with tanks. I also have thermal underwear from skiing and hiking trips. I'll be warm enough."

I felt confident staying in the cabin with a working fireplace. In the back of my mind crept a thought about a travel trailer. Frieda, Ben and I had gone earlier in the day to see the advertised trailer. It was in bad condition and therefore a no brainer; that particular trailer was not for me.

Larry continued showing me paperwork and explained he had papers in folders with keys taped to directions. He looked serious.

"In past years I hid certain things in our cabin for unexpected emergencies, which is why there is secrecy. Nothing is of much monetary value; it was just better than stuffing things in a mattress. You do know that's what some people did, don't you, Nancy?"

He looked at me with a sly grin.

"Yes in the old west that's how they did things, I get it." I matched his sly grin.

"The maps are not just directions to the cabin. They maps show the locations of certain hidden items."

Larry had carefully taped the keys to each map in question so the keys would not get lost. It felt like a treasure hunt to me. One of the requests on the folders looked very special and separated out from the other folders. Maybe it would be big safety deposits box in their Strawberry cabin.

"We trust the banks in Phoenix, but a small town like Strawberry, they don't even have a bank; at least not in the recent past. Maybe now. I don't know."

Larry knew a lot of old timers in Strawberry, even a few who lived there year round.

"The old timers are getting up in years and I just don't want to disturb any of them if I have a choice. I can ask them you know, Nancy but you are a better choice."

Besides making me feel young his comments indicated his level of trust in me. It confirmed our friendship, which was a warm and fuzzy. He was very dedicated to his wife, which I admired.

We both laughed again. I could sense Larry's sorrow. And at the same time his anxiety about Beth and her condition had to be on his mind.

"I am cool with everything you've given me Larry so far. Are you planning on returning tonight or tomorrow to the hospital?"

"I'm going to call after you leave; probably I'll sleep and go early tomorrow morning."

"Do you have a cell phone in case I need to call you and you are at the hospital?"

"No."

"Oh well I will just try and call the room if I need to reach you and you aren't at home."

Of course there was a possibility of Beth still being in the Intensive Care Unit. "Here's my cell number." And I handed him a card with my number on it. "Call me anytime and leave a message if you want. You know Larry I don't always have my cell turned on so just leave me a message if I don't answer okay?"

Larry nodded.

"You know I probably will stay up there for two or three days. Heck I might stop in Payson for a day or two on the way back. Are you in hurry for me to do these things?"

"No, I am grateful you are doing them for me, it means a lot, take your time." Larry had a tear in his eye and we hugged.

"If you think of anything else I need to know just call me." We hugged again and I saw his tears.

"You will never know how much I appreciate this, Nancy."

I pulled the folders close to my chest. He closed the front door behind me and I slowly walked next door to my house. Before I reached my door the moon caught my attention and I was instantly mesmerized.

Something about the moon was a prayer for me. The moon was so bright and drew my attention without question. Sunsets were beautiful and full of color and beauty but the moon in one iridescent glow was power.

Once inside my house I set aside the folders and poured myself a glass of Merlot. I decided to review the papers the next day, but for now I was enjoying some relaxation.

I changed into my pajamas and checked to make sure the tape recorder for taping my dreams was on my nightstand. This night would be a perfect time to remember a dream. My cat Tweetie jumped up on the bed. I petted her and told her I was leaving soon for a couple of days to Strawberry. Tweetie curled up and prepared to sleep. I was so grateful for such wonderful neighbors and friends. My neighbor JJ down the street would feed Tweetie. If JJ or I went out of town then the other would feed the pets. Mentally I prepared a list of things to do the next day; call JJ to feed Tweetie was first on my list of to dos. I turned off the bedroom light, finished my wine, and watched a little of David Letterman. In my mind floated my reoccurring theme of freedom in retirement.

Sleep came easily. I wasn't sure if it was the glass of wine or just plain old tiredness.

Chapter 15

Be Safe

No surprise, next morning I decided to head for the healing mountain or Thunderbird Mountain. It would be my last hike before heading to Strawberry. It was a quick drive to the mountain and it wasn't crowded. Actually only four cars were in the lot. I was twenty minutes into the hike when I looked up and saw Ted descending.

"Nancy, how are you doing?"

"Great I'm glad you are here Ted, I am leaving for Strawberry day after tomorrow. I'm going to check on a cabin for a friend. I'll probably be gone for a week."

Ted raised his eyebrows.

"Why now? In winter? Wouldn't it be better in spring? It's beautiful in Phoenix, why would you head to Strawberry, its cold up there?" Ted was right and I preferred spring, but my friend Larry needed me to go now. Besides it sounded like a mystery and I loved a good mystery.

"Well, I'm helping my neighbor. His wife fell sick in the middle of last summer and they left Strawberry in a hurry. I'm going to tie up some loose ends for them. Actually she is in the hospital now."

"Are you going with anyone? Want some company?"

"Thanks for the offer Ted, but I can handle it." It would be interesting to spend time with Ted off the mountain. Had it been a day trip I would have considered it. Besides Ted was a married man. His offer was genuinely kind but I wasn't sure how his wife would view it. It became irrelevant anyway.

"Be safe. The mountain will miss your nurturing presence Nancy."

I laughed and we hugged. He continued down and I continued up. I contemplated Ted's words "be safe" and I wondered if he was concerned about my safety or wanted time with me. I wished I had asked. Next time I would be quicker and ask. While I hiked I asked myself if I was afraid of going alone or being cold in the cabin. The rational side of my brain always had an answer like there was a fireplace and it would all work out. I made a mental note to check on the wood supply when I got to the cabin. And to bring a lot indoors so I wouldn't have to go outdoors in the middle of the night to get wood. It would also be a good idea to check on the nearest motel or hotel in case I got scared during the night. I could make a run to a motel and return to the cabin in daylight. I also wanted to check with Larry on the nearest neighbor.

When I reached the top of the mountain the view was clear with no smog. I could see the Indian Mountain, the one that looked like an Indian warrior looking up at the sky with a tear flowing down his cheek. Arizona was steeped in Indian history. I wished I knew more about the mystery of life. I knew some just knowing I could meditate. I could breathe in the breath of life or so I thought. Breath filled my lungs and brought all types of nourishment to my being. On the way down the mountain I prayed and said goodbye to the all the plants and animal life. I thought about Indian history and its impact on me. Everywhere I looked

I prayed. Under my breath I chanted "the God in me blesses the God in you; Namaste, Namaste." I felt very peaceful and gave a last glance to the mountain as I drove away. I was only leaving for a few days, maybe a week, and I already felt separation anxiety.

I opened my front door and glanced at my phone machine. No messages. I showered, changed clothes, and made lunch. I turned on the television and a show called "Starting Over" was on. I thought it was a great name for a show. There were two life coaches for several women starting over in a house. The women had been selected to live together and be exposed on television as they started their lives over from whatever had happened in the past. Some had been through divorce and some had death or a tragedy in their family. Both coaches were capable and compassionate women. It made me wonder if creating a new identity could fall under the Starting Over category. Instead of creating a new identity I could apply to be on the program as a new retiree. No, I thought not a good idea; retirement was a joy not a tragedy.

Hey, I could begin my new identity in Strawberry. I would be there a few days and it would give me practice. This was going to be double fun. It was a good thing I was traveling alone or my new identity would be blown. I laughed out loud. I must have some repressed spy who lived in my psyche.

Chapter 16

Folder Time

My plan was to leave the day after tomorrow. I decided to review Larry's folders and spread them across my dining room table, which Tweetie thought was an invitation to play. I picked her up and put her outside. All I needed was for Tweetie to mess up these papers. First I examined the directions to Strawberry and kept them separated from the other folders. The map showed the best way to reach Strawberry from Phoenix. I'd never been to Strawberry but it looked easy, even for me.

Next I looked for the directions to the cabin once I reached Strawberry. My concentration broke when the phone rang. It was Larry.

"Beth may not get out of the intensive care unit for a week, I thought I better let you know and see if you have any last minute questions. Are you leaving tomorrow or the next day?"

"I'm sorry about Beth, but you know she is well taken care of because that is a good hospital. I'll call you when I actually leave. I'm thinking day after tomorrow. How are you doing Larry?"

"Doing the best I can, another friend will be here shortly for moral support, but I wanted to know if you have any questions? I wasn't sure when you were going."

"I'll keep Beth in my prayers, actually both you and Beth. One question, how close is the nearest neighbor?"

"Across the street, but they are down here in Phoenix for the winter."

The closest occupied home that he knew was about a mile from his cabin. He gave me the name of the people but without a phone number. I wrote it down on the pad by my phone. The phone cradled in my ear fell to the floor.

"Sorry Larry I dropped the phone, give me a minute."

I could see the folders still stretched across my dining room table. Less than twenty feet from my dining room window Larry was probably sitting in his comfortable chair talking to me on the phone.

"I'm back."

"You can find all the phone numbers in the cabin in Strawberry; the drawer under the microwave in the kitchen has an address book with the numbers. Call the people first and stop by the house; they will be happy for company."

"I think I got it, I hope Beth feels better soon and remember, Larry, take care of you."

I hung up the phone and went for a chocolate bar.

I started feeling a little uneasy about being alone in an isolated cabin especially since Ted made a comment to me about my safety driving alone. I pulled out my AAA book for Arizona and looked for hotels or motels in Strawberry. The phone rang and it was Maggie, an old friend from work. We chatted awhile.

"Maggie want to go with me to Strawberry?"

Fear had gotten the best of me. I let Ted's comment of fear take root in my psyche. If Ted wasn't married we could have had fun hiking around Strawberry and figured out sleeping accommodations that were comfortable for each of us.

Maggie declined.

"I don't like Strawberry and I have company coming."

I was back to square one. I wished George were in town. He would have been game for adventure. He liked to hike and I was sure hiking would be bountiful in Strawberry. Oh well if I really wanted a new identity it would have to include me as a braver being. I could think of myself as fearless. A lot of women traveled alone. Many single women had handled ranches with livestock on their own. The song "Anything you can do I can do better" played in my head. Oh yes, this was going to be an adventure.

I thought of Oakley in Ohio near Cincinnati where my cousins were born and raised. It wasn't until I was an adult that I realized the town, Oakley, was named for Annie Oakley. She had been a strong unafraid woman. Strong women were nothing new to me. I came of age during bra burning and women's rights in a very conservative city. Many times I was the sole liberal in a room of conservatives. In those times my Irish heritage of debating came to the forefront. I loved to debate.

I returned my consciousness to the dining room table. I brought out the rest of the folders and found some colored markers in my desk. Each folder was labeled with some notes by Larry and included a key. Since I didn't know the contents of the various locked boxes I numbered the folders #1, #2, #3 etc. I was organized. I looked at the clock and it was after four pm. I was meeting friends for Mexican food across town at six. I gathered the stuff and put it in a neat pile. I told myself I would resume organizing later. I opened the back door and let Tweetie in. Someone had to guard the house while I was gone and that would be Tweetie.

"Tweetie you can earn your keep by being a watch cat."

I changed clothes and headed out the door for a light evening with friends.

Chapter 17

Here's to Strawberry

The next morning I woke up to the welcome sound of rain. I knew I had the whole day to pack and get ready for tomorrow's trip. My wardrobe for the trip would be comfortable jeans and sweatshirts. That was my normal attire for any trip. My goal was to leave around six in morning, which would give me daylight hours to check out things in Strawberry. It would also give me time to stop along the way if I wanted. I could look for a motel if it made me feel safer. My best guess was I'd be in a motel in Strawberry for most of the five days if I stayed that long.

I had the six folders that Larry made for me setting on my table. It was going to be like a treasure hunt. I could average completion of two folders a day if I wanted to stretch it, or I could possibly complete all six in one day and return to Phoenix. No, I was sure I wanted to spend a minimum of three days in Strawberry. Quaint old towns in Arizona were quickly becoming a thing of the past.

Enough thinking and out of my bed I gingerly arose and made my way to the dining room table. I started reviewing and organizing keys and papers. I didn't know what was in the boxes he wanted me to open. I concluded it must be important stuff. I knew I would bring back whatever it was he wanted me to deliver to him. I didn't want to ask a lot of questions. He had given me the keys and folders for a reason. If he didn't want me to open anything he wouldn't have given me the keys. Maybe I was finding family stuff in the boxes; like a will. I figured it was old people stuff. At some point soon I would also be an old person and this was what old people do. Right now I was in my fifties and I had plenty of time to be old later. My focus was on my trip to Strawberry.

I selected music and motivational CDs from my collection for the drive north. I checked my purse for my AAA card and planned to stop at the bank for cash. I was quite certain ATMs were everywhere but just in case. There had been two ATMs in the Grand Canyon so surely there would be one in Strawberry.

I let Tweetie outside and packed some clothes and toiletries. Then I went to the kitchen for any essentials I would need in the cabin. I negated that. It was doubtful I would stay in the cabin. For food I was sure there would be fast food. It is everywhere. If they had a gym or fitness center I could work out. That would be cool. I put hiking clothes in my suitcase in case I found a suitable mountain. Just maybe I might happen upon someone I knew or someone safe to hike with. The likelihood was slim to none, but I was an optimist. Taking on a new identity would entertain me. I planned to rationalize further on my drive to Strawberry. I gathered up the six folders with maps and keys and placed them in a cardboard box. It was a ratty box that I kept in the back of my car for important papers. These were important papers and the box was the right size. I would review them all in Strawberry. I would have more time.

I wanted to stop by the hospital to see Beth. I knew only family was allowed into Intensive Care so it was not a good option. The rest of the day was uneventful. I went to bed early so as to wake up early. Tweetie knew something was up. I knew that JJ would take good care of her. Tweetie would be well fed.

Chapter 18

Time to Go

The next morning came quickly and the alarm was ringing at five thirty am. Five thirty in the morning is brutal. I decided I didn't want an alarm clock for the trip. My watch would be just fine. I recalled a dream last night but not much of the detail.

I was on the same mountainside as from the previous dream. There were rocks all around me and my attention was focused on rocks moving.

My interpretation was minimal. The mountain was telling me I didn't know the power of individual rocks on the mountain trail because the rocks were moving. Then I recalled they vibrated. Vibration was energy in movement. I didn't know what, if anything, it meant. Maybe there was unrealized power all around me like vibrating rocks. I tape recorded the dream and got out of bed. My day was started.

Breakfast was quick and my car was packed. I was grateful for my organizational skills. All I had to do was get in the car and drive off. The car was full of gas and ready to go. I gave Tweetie a quick pet and headed out the door. I said a prayer for a safe drive. I knew I had guardian angels and I kept them busy. Guardian angels were one of the things I was most grateful for from my Catholic education. I felt a protecting angelic presence and it was the nuns who taught me to call the presence guardian angels. It was a delightful teaching. I wondered if they still taught that. I had worked in public schools and there was never a mention of God or religion. Not talking about God would have seemed very strange to a younger me. Nonetheless here I was driving to Strawberry by myself with my guardian angels. It was all perception. Traffic was slow and it was still somewhat dark outside. A lot of trucks were on the road. I didn't mind trucks; I was retired and could take my time. Following a truck was an option.

I put a Wayne Dyer CD "The Power of Intention" into the CD player. I listened to his words that inspired me to set my intentions for the day. My intentions were to be helpful to Larry, to arrive safely in Strawberry, and to create a new identity for a couple of days. I could do all three. I knew the mind was powerful. People had talked about affirmations for years. I heard a million times the Ernest Holmes quote "change your thinking change your life." The first time it was quoted to me it was from a Science of Mind textbook. Almost every time I mentioned the source of the quote as Science of Mind or Ernest Holmes people cringed and thought it was Scientology and no, it wasn't. Generally the conversation turned to self-fulfilled prophecy. One would think something over and over and it came true. Another way I heard it "As a Man Thinketh." Initially, I learned the most from the negative side because it grabbed my attention. My negativity forced me to question myself as to how I got in the mess. I probably downplayed positive occurrences as accidents. I sure have changed. Now I don't even believe in accidents. People generally agreed that in their own experiences their thoughts impacted their life. The power of thought could be harnessed for good or negative. One of my spiritual teachers taught me to set an egg timer for five minutes and as it ticked I'd write down every thought that came into my head. I did it. It was shocking how badly I talked to myself in the five-minute time. It was years ago and I still remember. If I did that exercise again today the percentage of negative self-talk would significantly be decreased. Without question I knew my self-talk was more positive.

I was thinking too much. Music would be soothing. I flipped to radio. I came upon oldies music and started singing along. Singing was always good for getting my energy up. The drive from Phoenix to Payson was soothing compared to the ride from Phoenix to Flagstaff. I-17 from Phoenix to Flagstaff was a typical interstate road. The Beeline Highway to Payson was curvy and changes in the desert elevation were visible. The low to high desert shifted from cactus to tall pine trees. Wildflowers blanketed the drive in spring. It was mostly a drive with nature and very few structures, some businesses and a sprinkling of residences. One huge castle-type building, a casino, stood out like a sore thumb. Part of my drive went through reservation land. Tribes owned all the casinos in Arizona.

Route 87 would take me all the way into Strawberry. It went through Payson. Larry had a copy of a *Payson Rim Country Relocation Guide* that he had tucked in with the folders. It gave a history of the Payson area/ Mogollon Rim that I had read with my morning coffee.

The first inhabitants of this area were an ancient people called the Mogollons-named for Juan Ignacia Flores Mogollon, a Spanish colonial governor. Later the Apache Indians moved into the area. The first white man to inhabit the area was during the Civil War. Fort McDowell, Camp Reno and Camp Verde were established in the event the Confederate Army invaded. After the Civil War they stayed on to protect against the Apache Indians.

After hearing stories from soldiers it was believed that gold and silver were to be found in the area. About 40 miners came hoping to strike it rich. When very little of these minerals were found, they decided to stay on anyway to become ranchers and loggers. In 1882 the town was incorporated as Union Park. However the locals continued to call it Green Valley. In 1884 a post office was established and was called Payson – for Senator Louis Payson (Congressional Chairman of Post Offices and Post Roads).

The Woolsey Expedition came through the Pine area in 1864. They called the mountains the Penal Mountains – mispronouncing the Apache word for deer- Pinal. Despite much strife and unbearable hardships the Mormons settled this area in 1879.

Strawberry was first called Strawberry Valley (for the abundance of wild strawberries growing there.) The Strawberry Schoolhouse was established in 1884. It was a one-room schoolhouse made from logs. The school was no longer used after 1916, but it may still be visited today.

I made a mental note to visit the schoolhouse. Route 87 wasn't crowded but there were lots of trucks and motor homes. Back in the seventies when I drove on Route 87 it was a two-lane highway. We had been stuck behind a semi and crawled up the highway. Now it was four-lane and quite smooth. I could see the layers of color as I approached Payson and the Mogollon Rim. The Relocation Guide described the Rim.

The Mogollon Rim according to Arizona Highways is "Arizona's Mighty Backbone" and meanders for over 200 miles. It is made up of sedimentary plateau rocks deposited on each other in the Paleozoic Age. It has an average height of 7,000 feet.

It sounded like some great hiking country not to mention the forest of trees. I did some of my best thinking driving in a car. I still didn't like driving, but I made the best of it. I flipped back in consciousness to my life as a teenager. I imagined what I, as a teen, might think about who I was today. Some of my judgments were positive and some negative. I knew that as an adult my life to this point was a tapestry. It fit together.

My memory surfaced another teacher whose words echoed in my mind; "if you knew better you would have done better." I questioned that teacher as to why I didn't know better. Most of us are more judgmental of ourselves than we are of other people. I learned the Golden Rule in grammar school; do unto others, as you would have them do unto you. I had a teacher who once said if people treated others as badly as we treat ourselves than no one would be talking to anybody. That was a sad thought but somewhat true nonetheless. I caught myself thinking; if I have become more real and less negative through the years then so have many other people. The consciousness of society had to have grown as well even though there were still wars and crap. Enough, I needed a diversion to bring me back to positive and creative.

My new identity, now that was worth some time. I could choose an identity of being loving and supportive in all relationships including with me. The spiritual aspect of me was not in need. It was complete unto self. It was the emotional, mental, and thinking parts of me that needed help. In other words my human parts needed help. I felt an intention bubble to the surface. Yes, my intention was to be loving and supportive in all my relationships. I wondered if that would feel different than my regular self. Yes, I need a new name to fully capture this new intention for my identity.

The sound of a loud truck horn honking pierced my thoughts. It brought my attention fully to the road and I could see an accident up ahead. Lights of a police cruiser flashed and an ambulance approached the scene. Several people sat on the side of the road and appeared to be from the cars involved in the wreck. One lady had a bloody arm. Car damage looked minimal. That was good, no one looked badly injured. I inched past at a slow pace. My stomach was growling. It was either hunger or anxiety. Either way I decided to stop at the next decent looking restaurant. I liked to be waited on. If I didn't find one I had a reserve of granola bars and apples in the cooler. Coolers were a great invention. Throw in some ice, drinks, and food all together and a person had a back up food plan.

Views on the Beeline Highway were beautiful with massive tall pine trees and rugged desert terrain. The temperatures cooled as the elevation changed. The elevation in Strawberry would be six thousand feet, much higher than Phoenix. I was a true Phoenician because cold energized me. Cold weather was welcomed after a long hot summer. The only problem was Phoenician blood thinned out as a result of heat. I would need extra clothes to keep me warm in the colder climate. I enjoyed wearing sweaters and it was seldom that I had the pleasure of donning one in Phoenix. I hated sweaters that pulled over my head. I wore blazers or cardigans. As a post menopausal woman I was usually warm and layering clothes was my best solution. It was the only realistic solution. I learned it was easier to unbutton a cardigan and throw it over my shoulders that it was to continually pull a sweater up and down over my head. Cardigans were most convenient.

Chapter 19

Beginnings

I saw an orange Denny's Restaurant sign to the left side of the highway about five hundred feet ahead. It looked okay. I knew Denny's had a veggie burger and great onion rings even though the rings made me gassy. No one would care if I was gassy as I was alone. It was about eleven when I looked at my watch. I was that much closer to Strawberry. I turned into Denny's lot and parked right in front of the door to the restaurant. Parking in front was convenient and I could keep an eye on my car. The hostess greeted me and introduced herself as Sally. She tucked a pencil behind her ear.

"What's your name, honey?"

"Annie." I said confidently.

"How many in your party, Annie?"

"One, just me."

Sally graciously led me to a booth and I sat. She handed me a menu and motioned to a waiter.

"Annie, this is your server Bill, he will take your order when you are ready. Enjoy your meal."

Bill had a deadpan expression, but raised his pencil to his order pad.

"What would you like to drink?"

"Iced tea."

This was fun and I was thrilled. I was Annie. I was someone else who no one knew. I wondered if I was obvious about something being different, maybe a smirk on my face or a look of surprise. No one knew and no one cared. I hadn't consciously thought to say Annie. It was quick. My subconscious spat up Annie. I was sure it related somehow to Annie Oakley. I reminded myself that my intention for this new identity as Annie was to be supportive and loving. I may have stated it as loving and supportive. The order of the words didn't matter, just as it didn't matter if I was Annie or Nancy. I was going to eat. Bill returned with his order pad.

"Annie, what can I get you?"

"I think I'll have a veggie burger and onion rings."

"Coming right up." Bill left.

Lunch was good and best of all quick. I paid my bill with cash and left a nice tip for Bill. After all, Annie was loving and supportive. It would have been a hoot if I had charged my lunch on a card that read Nancy. I doubted if anyone would have noticed. Sally might have noticed. I stopped in the bathroom and as an after thought counted my cash. I had one hundred and seventy dollars in cash. I tucked it back in my purse and headed out the front door. Sally and Bill both waved.

"Bye, Annie."

I left Denny's with a smile from ear to ear. I made a mental note to eat at this same place on the way home just to hear if someone would call me Annie. The rest of my drive to Strawberry was smooth and the highway was lined with more beautiful trees.

It was like driving down an old-fashioned country road. Yeah, I could hear John Denver in my mind singing Country Roads. My hand fell to the passenger side of my car and rested upon my Nikon camera. It was a fancy digital camera. My judgment of myself was that I had wasted money purchasing it. I told myself at the time that I would use it a lot, which I didn't. Tomorrow I would take pictures of the cabin and whatever else struck my fancy. The more I used it and learned how to use it, the happier I became about the purchase. I thought about purchasing a smaller lighter weight camera for my backpack and keeping this for real photo jobs.

The sign read Strawberry two miles and I was glad. My back was getting tired of sitting and I wanted to be settled. Strawberry was not listed in their tour book. It was going to be a very small town. I had phoned AAA for recommendations and they had given me two names of lodges. Both lodges had available rooms or at least they did when I called from Phoenix. I wondered if they would be like most hotels and require a charge card as I checked in. I hadn't made a reservation just an inquiry into availability so no one knew my name. The rates were roughly sixty dollars a night. I didn't have enough to pay in cash and register as Annie. How silly was that anyway, it was just a name. Trying on new ideas was part of retirement. Annie was me, in a different way. Annie was retired Nancy. I knew if I really wanted to check in as Annie I could find cash, as there had to be ATMs in Strawberry. I laughed at myself. I actually debated with myself if I should check in as Nancy or Annie. I drove around both motels and decided that the Strawberry Lodge was clearly a better-looking place. And beside cleanliness there was a carving of an angel over the door. Strawberry Lodge it was. Before I pulled in I caught a glimpse of an ATM sign over what looked like the old general store. It was tempting to get cash and sign in as Annie, but Annie and my car license plate wouldn't match if anyone bothered to check.

Chapter 20

The Strawberry Lodge

I entered the lobby, which was a bar. There was no front desk sign so I asked at the restaurant counter next to the bar. That was the check in area. The Strawberry Lodge was built in 1962. It was quite rustic with heads of elk, old pictures, and other antiquities. I asked for a second floor non-smoking room with a view if they had it. All of the rooms had views. This was Strawberry with an elevation of six thousand feet. It was a never ending forest of trees. The clerk gave me a key for room 207 and a map of the local area. I remembered to ask about other restaurants in town, which wasn't too productive since I was standing in their restaurant. They informed me that the ATM at the old general store was not functional. The thought of asking about movie theaters in town crossed my mind, but I had brought a lot of books to read in case I got bored at night. This was going to be exciting I decided and I was up for it. I retrieved my luggage from the car and headed to my room. The room was fairly plain; definitely a no frills old-fashioned spot. There was a small balcony and a tiny bathroom. The view was all I could want it to be. If I was here to journal or write it would be perfect. I sat on the bed and pulled out the maps of the town and the map Larry had given me. It took me about twenty minutes to figure out where I was and where the cabin was on the map.

Taking a nap became an option and I did. This was a mini vacation. I opened the curtains and saw this landscape of green, red, and brown. As far as I could see there were trees; sequoia, pine, pinion, cottonwood, mesquite, and palo verde. It was a forest of trees and color. I opened the window and breathed in fresh cold air. My lungs loved it. I closed the window and laid down for a nap. My brain was too stimulated. Rather than waste time I got up and got into the car. Driving around town to familiarize myself satisfied my need to know exactly where I was. I had my map and camera, a true tourist. In a blink of an eye I was out of town or at least off the main highway. Strawberry only had one main road. I passed a sign for the old schoolhouse but decided to save it for another day. After a while I found the turnoff for Larry's cabin. This was cause for celebration; it was too easy. Before I knew it I was three miles down the road looking for my next turnoff to Larry's. In the distance I saw an elderly gentleman wearing a cowboy hat walking his dog along the unpaved road. The man and I exchanged waves because that was what people did in small towns. I bet he could tell stories and might even know Larry and Beth. I was glad I had a jeep with four-wheel drive. Four-wheel drive had gotten me out of many jams. However I needed to be careful, as tonight was not a good time to get into a jam. I barely knew where I was. In a flash I remembered to be loving and supportive of myself, which was something Annie would have suggested. My cell phone was back in the lodge so it was a good supportive decision to return to the lodge. I was happy that I had a better idea of where I would be driving the following day. The sun went down early in Arizona winters and even though it was only five pm it was getting dark. I gave a sigh of relief as I turned the car around and drove back to town.

The onion rings I had for lunch began to kick in and upset my stomach. Soup and salad sounded like a good dinner. I parked in the lodge parking lot and entered their dining area. There were three rooms in the dining area, the bar, and two dining rooms. One of the dining rooms had a counter with stools. It was all casual. It looked rustic and full of character. A woman in cowgirl clothing greeted me.

"Come on in" she waved to me. "Sit wherever you like." She handed me a menu.

"Thanks."

It wasn't too crowded so I sat at a booth by a window. The window looked out on the main street, the only street through town. A couple came in and glanced at me with a smile. I returned the smile. A couple of young cowboy looking guys came in; it was all you could eat taco night. Several more people came in for the tacos. Not me. I ordered vegetable soup and a cranberry chicken salad. It was fun watching people who I decided were locals. Each one had a story in their face. I concluded people who lived in Strawberry for the winter were extremely strong.

After my non-eventful dinner I returned to my room and pulled out my cell phone to check for messages. I had called Larry before I left so he knew I was on my way to Strawberry. There were no messages. I hooked up my phone to the battery charger. I was known for ignoring my cell phone. I only turned it on if I was expecting a call or if I had an emergency. Several times in my travels I have had to call AAA for roadside assistance.

Once inside my room at the lodge I double locked the door and turned on the TV. Before I could count to six I fell asleep.

Chapter 21

The Cabin

Sometime late at night I heard a door slam. My eyes opened and stared right into the ceiling light that blazed into my eyes. It had been on all night. I was startled and then remembered I was in Strawberry, Arizona at the Strawberry Lodge. Doors slamming are a natural sound in any motel. I was not the only guest. I got up and changed into my pajamas. The bedside clock read one thirty am. My guess was that the motel guest who slammed the door probably closed the local bar. My teeth brushed I returned to bed and put my tape recorder on the nightstand. In case I woke up remembering a dream I could talk it into the tape recorder.

My head hit the pillow and the next thing I knew it was morning. There was a whole chorus of doors that opened and closed. I got ready for the day; completed a fifteen-minute meditation, and set my intention. The Strawberry Lodge, I discovered, had a continental breakfast, which included great coffee. Before leaving the room I took the extra roll of toilet paper in case I got stuck somewhere or there wasn't any at the cabin. My cell phone was in my purse and I felt like Nancy Drew in one of her mystery novels. As a teenager back in the fifties I had read all of her books and, of course, I felt a connection since we were both named Nancy.

Once outside I felt the coldness and was grateful for my winter coat. The thought of snow crossed my mind. I couldn't remember the last time I had driven in snow. My estimated drive time to the cabin was thirty minutes because of the dirt roads and unknown conditions. Now that I was awake and in bright daylight driving around, I sensed the sweetness of a small town; kind of like a fairy tale. It was picture perfect and I had my camera. Before I could count to ten I was out of my car. My camera clicked. Everywhere I looked was beauty. As far as my eye could see was a multitude of colors, mostly green, from all types of trees, pine, pinion, cottonwood, oak etc. The sky was blue with large fluffy clouds. What struck me most was the clean air, no signs of pollution. It gave crystal clear a new meaning. My pictures were great and I could print them on my new computer program when I got back to Phoenix. Ben and Frieda had given me a photo print program for Christmas last year. I could experiment with these images. My red jeep looked so cool in the mountains next to all the tall green trees. The chili pepper red color of my Jeep was hard to miss in the midst of green and brown. With all these trees I thought maybe I would see a tree nymph like the one I had painted, framed and hung over my fireplace in Phoenix. I looked, but never saw one on my healing mountain. Maybe one would be here in Strawberry.

Back in the car I continued my drive and I figured I was within fifteen minutes to the cabin. Up ahead I saw the same older man wearing a cowboy hat and walking his dog on a side path. He must know Larry and Beth. It crossed my mind to contact some of the names in Larry's phone book. I decided against it since I didn't need additional information, but it could be interesting. I seemed to know where I was going. Actually there weren't too many turnoffs to confuse me. Cabins that I passed were looking more like houses, but they were spread out by any city standard. My house in Phoenix was only 1,200 square feet. Some people in big homes had bedrooms that size. In the darkness of night I was glad my place was small. Large houses have lots of strange noises. Houses or cabins were few and far between up here.

I rounded the twentieth bend and up ahead on the right was Larry and Beth's cabin.

"Cabin" I shouted out loud "it is a big ole house! Oh wow!" The driveway circled behind the cabin so I drove in and pulled around to the back door. I turned off the car engine and just immersed myself in the stillness and beauty.

After about ten minutes I picked up my purse and the box with all the folders. I felt very official with this box tucked under my arm. It must be an old social worker thing of mine. The key and papers for opening the door were in the top orange folder. Unlike my home in Phoenix there was no burglar alarm that needed to be turned off. There was a top and bottom lock. To my amazement both locks opened smoothly and I was inside the cabin.

The cabin was meticulous with just a few things left out on counters. It was neater than I had left my house. I entered one extraordinarily large room with several side doors leading to who knows where. The kitchen was part of the large room and central to it all was a huge fireplace. The all brick fireplace was large and spectacular. I could almost smell burnt wood coming from it. I had a fireplace at home that was tiny by comparison. If I could figure out the flu handle on this fireplace then I'd have a fire in it just for the day. Larry had suggested that I sleep here but I had chickened out. I didn't feel comfortable in a strange cabin in a strange location. The strangeness was melting quickly because of the rustic beauty inside and outside this place. I could certainly understand why Larry and Beth had spent the past thirty summers in this cabin. It was quiet and reverent. All I could hear was the rustle of wind. Every window had a view. I felt alone, not a scared alone, but aloneness immersed in beauty.

I thought to myself about all the towns, villages, and countries that existed on this planet. I was too focused on my life in

Phoenix and needed expansion. The earth was full of beauty. I questioned myself as to why I hadn't ever been to Strawberry or taken more short trips in Arizona. Through the years Larry and Beth had invited me to visit them anytime in their cabin, but I had never found the time. There it was again the echo resounding in my brain, my old motto "when I get time." Ah the mystery of freedom that is retirement. Finally the time was here and the place was now. The mind was so interesting in all its creativity. It couldn't be anything less. I stopped and stared out the open door at the wonders of nature.

There were big cushions on the floor and lots of chairs. I chose a kitchen chair and began spreading the folders on the table. Either I could process all the folders right now or do them one at a time on separate days. Spread over the days the tasks would cover my whole visit. I was retired and not in a hurry. I had hurried my whole life to get everything done. God only knows what I had missed in my hurry. Larry knew I was making a mini vacation out of this trip so he wasn't in any hurry or expecting anything from me anytime soon. I loved freedom. It was sacred to me being in someone's residence and knowing that they trusted me implicitly with very private information. Anyway Larry trusted me. Beth had been sick. I doubted she had the capacity to know I was in their cabin. As I did with most things I sat in meditation and said a prayer for wisdom and guidance in achieving my goals here in the cabin. I felt supportive and loving toward Larry, Beth and most certainly for myself.

"Annie would be proud" I laughed out loud "and Nancy is pretty cool too".

Even though it was still early in the afternoon it was too late for a wood burning fire. It would have taken too long to ensure the fire was totally out before I left. I looked for some candles; I had old matches in my purse. The door over the refrigerator looked like a good place to keep candles.

"Yes, candles."

There was a vanilla and an unscented candle. I lit them both and gave myself a tour of the cabin. I had almost forgotten the folders, almost. The tour occupied my mind. There were two small bedrooms, two bathrooms, a master bedroom with half bath and large walk-in linen closet. My favorite space was the huge room I had entered and for lack of a better name called it the great room. All doors were off the great room. It was well equipped with a television and a working phone. I hadn't even thought to ask Larry if the cabin had a working phone. He probably forgot to have it disconnected for winter. The kitchen had all modern conveniences and lots of frozen food. It was probably better equipped than my house in Phoenix. Sometimes I questioned if older people, especially Larry and Beth, ate appropriately. A lot of people lost their appetites as they aged. Larry was the chef and food shopper. He had been doing it for going on three years. Beth was physically challenged especially after her bout with Shingles. Larry had this kitchen well stocked. A person could live quite well in this cabin for several months.

The cabin was chilly and I knew I didn't want to fool with a propane tank. I continued looking around. As I would have guessed there were floor to ceiling bookcases. In the past Larry and I had many philosophical conversations. Beth was not as vocal as Larry and she had become even less vocal in the last few years. I glanced at the books on the shelves and realized I was familiar with most of them. Several I had never even heard of before seeing them on the shelf. All the titles appealed to me with most in the philosophical or religious realm. I flipped through Walden Pond. Suddenly I became aware of a rustling sound outside. It frightened

me. I peered through the kitchen window and I was eye-to-eye with
a coyote that looked hungry and cold. I spooked the animal and he
took off. It was definitely chilly inside and outside it was beginning
to cloud up. I brought the vanilla candle closer and curled up on
the floor with a cushion and opened up Walden Pond. Years ago in
the sixties or seventies I had read it cover to cover. In the seventies
I had kept a copy of it my Volkswagen Thing for those occasions
in the desert when I wanted inspiration. A couple of hours flew
by. My stomach growled. I found a granola bar in my purse and
crunched on it. I paused from reading and contemplated how my
life journey had brought me to this point; it was very peaceful and
free. I couldn't figure out if feeling peaceful or free came first. I
certainly could not be peaceful if I wasn't free. And I couldn't be
free if I wasn't peaceful. The words meant different things to me
and I loved them both.

I was getting sleepy and decided to head back to town for a
nice warm home cooked dinner at the lodge. I rationalized that
the earlier I went to sleep the earlier I could return. If I arrived
early enough the next morning I could build a fire. I gathered my
unread folders and put them back in the box to take to the car.
The folders would be good reading material over dinner. Without
a dinner companion reading was a very welcome option. I blew
out the candles and locked both doors. The jeep started right up
and I was grateful for the heater in my car. I snapped a couple of
pictures of the cabin and was off down the bumpy back road. The
drive back was pleasant. I stopped by my motel room to freshen
up before dinner.

Chapter 22

Folder Review Again

As I entered the dining room I envisioned mashed potatoes, gravy, fried chicken, green beans, and a garden salad. This was the ranking order of my comfort foods. People in the dining room seemed a little friendlier than last night. The waitress remembered me. People waved as if they knew me. Maybe I was friendlier. I was probably more comfortable since it was my second night in a row eating and sleeping at the same place. I could have passed as a regular in here as I was on my healing mountain. I imagined a lot of people passed through Strawberry on their way to somewhere else. I was anything but inconspicuous. At five feet ten inches tall I was hard to miss. I appreciated all the pleasantries, which made me feel like a local. But no one asked my name as they had at Denny's. I wasn't even sure how much information I would volunteer if anyone asked. Traveling alone one had to be careful. Some day I may want to come back as Annie. Instead of going through the folders as I had planned I read the local newspaper. I didn't want to miss anything exciting that might be in town even though I thought that what I was doing was pretty darn exciting. I ate everything I ordered. The food was definitely home cooked. I felt nourished, paid the bill and returned to my room.

Back in my room with the TV on, I pulled out the box of folders I had dragged around with me all day. I marked the orange folder, #1, mission accomplished; it had the map and key to the cabin. There were five folders left. The next folder, #2, was green. I opened it and it contained directions for locating titles for Larry's land and cabin. Larry had neatly taped a little key in the upper right hand corner and, of course. The instructions led to a book safe hidden on the third shelf behind a non-descript book title. Book safes if I recalled correctly appeared to look like a book but were hollow inside. I was surprised I hadn't observed something odd when I rummaged through the books on the shelves. Tomorrow it would be a piece of cake finding the title. Larry's paperwork indicated it was a copy of a title and not the original. It made me question why a copy needed to hidden. I knew Larry and Beth had owned their cabin for years.

The next folder, #3, was blue and it too had a key neatly taped in the upper right hand corner. This time I read the key opened a wall safe with personal papers inside. This was interesting. It was in a separate place from the titles. Titles were important pieces of paper and you would think it would be with his personal papers. Maybe the original title was with his personal papers in the wall safe. It was clear I needed to review these papers with Larry. Maybe it was better because I would have had lots of questions and it was none of my business anyway. I rationalized that none of the papers were too important because there was no rush. Larry made it sound as if he normally closed out the cabin at the end of each summer and then reopened it in summer. Maybe he took all this stuff back and forth with him each time. He was rushed when he left the cabin last time because of Beth's health. I could just imagine Larry sorting and packing summer clothes for Strawberry and winter clothes for Phoenix. I could see moving clothes back and forth but moving papers, if he did, was questionable. People had their habits and rituals, besides I didn't own anything of importance other than my home and it was where I could be found ninety-five percent of the time. I was a homebody. If I was lucky enough to ever own two homes then it could be a different story and a different set of responsibilities. That might be nice.

Folder #4 was white and its key was to a storage locker. The folder contained a map of where the shed was on the grounds. I vaguely recollected seeing a shed on the premises when I was there. I thought I could see it in my mind's eye. If I remembered correctly it was a run of the mill shed. I guessed Larry gave me this key to the shed in case I need something like a hammer, a wrench or maybe garden tools. It made sense if I had stayed in the cabin then I may have needed some tools. I bet there was a riding lawn mower in that shed and sure enough there on the map was a little drawing of a sit down mower in the back corner. As I looked closer to Larry's directions I saw a red arrow pointing to what looked like a weed eater. Larry was directing me to bring the weed eater back to Phoenix. I got it. This was making more sense now.

The fifth folder, #5, was red and its key was to open something by the basement. Wow, I wished I could remember anything Larry may have told me when he gave me these folders. Larry was a very intelligent, emotional guy who was very concerned about his wife. I sensed he thought the end for Beth might be near. He had confided to several of us that it was getting progressively harder and harder for him to care for her. Larry was somewhat frail and a hundred and ten pounds wet. All one hundred and ten pounds were dedicated to his Beth. I knew how meticulous Larry was and that whatever he had written for directions was complete. I was glad, in retrospect, that I hadn't bothered him with a lot of unnecessary questions. Again I reminded myself that I wasn't picking up anything of major importance. If Beth weren't in the hospital, I probably wouldn't have been asked or volunteered. If the children lived closer they would have gladly volunteered.

Chapter 23

A Fire in the Fireplace

My eyes were shutting and I decided to change into my pajamas. I had requested a wake up call for six am. That will give me plenty of time to meditate, shower and be on the road by seven. I could have that fireplace blazing by nine or ten at the latest. The fire could be phased out by four, putting my return to the lodge by six pm. It was a good plan. For the umpteenth time I put all the folders back in the box. I made a mental note to finish the last folder on whatever day in front of a roaring fire at the cabin. No matter what tomorrow morning there would be a fire in the fireplace. With a warmed heart I looked forward to the new day.

My stay in Strawberry could be extended. When I checked in I had told them four nights. I could be finished tomorrow retrieving this folder/key stuff for Larry and on Thursday either relax or head home. My preference would be to stay and relax. Four nights was my original plan for my mini-vacation, but of course, three nights would be cheaper. I fluctuated and settled on taking my time. Retired folk have no need to hurry. Larry had offered to pay my lodging bill, but I wouldn't allow it. It was my decision to stay at the lodge rather than in his cabin. Maybe some other time in the future, if he invited me to the cabin , I would accept. But for now I turned off all the lights in my room and focused on a good nights sleep. I knew it would all fall into place, it always did. That was my intention.

The next thing I consciously knew was the phone ringing and it was my wake up call. It was six am. I showered, dressed warmly and threw extra granola bars into my purse. The continental breakfast offered in the motel was just fine because the coffee was great. I got into my jeep and was off. I noticed a light dusting of snow on the ground and it seemed colder, but I would be okay because I was well bundled. I turned on my car heater and thought, with pleasure, about building a fire when I got to the cabin. No time to stop for pictures I wanted to get that fireplace going.

I made the first familiar turn on the side road and there in the middle of nowhere was the same man I had seen yesterday walking his dog. We waved to each other and smiled. Behind the man on the road I saw smoke curling out of a chimney in a distant cabin. It probably was his cabin. I was grateful that I had noticed another cabin in use. I wasn't alone. It was definitely a colder day than yesterday. After a couple of miles I entered the driveway to Larry's cabin. The driveway wrapped behind the cabin and I pulled all the way to the back. The first folder, the orange one I reminded myself, contained the door key. I pulled out the key and unlocked both locks and entered the cabin with ease, just as I had yesterday. The inside of the cabin was just as beautiful today as I had found it yesterday. Everything was just as I had left it. My eyes landed on the fireplace and there was plenty of wood next to it. After I had fumbled a minute or two the flu opened. The wood was stacked in a neat pile with plenty of old newspapers on the side. I crumbled some paper under the grate and placed the wood on top. I stroked the match, smelled the sulfur, ignited the paper, put my feet up, and sat back in pure joy. All the comforts of home.

After drinking all that morning coffee I needed to use the bathroom. In hiking I had no problem going to the bathroom behind bushes. Instead of using the bushes I felt brave and was going to locate the water valve to bring water into the house. My bravery paid off and the water flowed in the pipes to the cabin. Having a bathroom was a luxury.

Smoke billowed up my chimney and I was very content. I picked up the Walden book from yesterday and began reading where I had left off. I lost focus on the book because my mind kept returning to my purpose for being at the cabin. It wasn't to read Walden Pond. Again I dug through the box with the folders. I got busy locating the things Larry wanted me to bring back to Phoenix.

First I found the book safe right where Larry indicated it would be. I removed what looked like a yellowing old envelope with a faded yellow ribbon. Interesting, I thought, and placed the old envelop inside the green folder. I carefully re-taped the key to the upper corner. Mission accomplished. I wished I had thought to bring fresh tape with me. Then again there was probably some in the cabin somewhere. I rummaged through the kitchen drawers. Sure enough there it was and two packages of it at that. It was amazing how well new versus old tape adhered to paper. I pondered unfolding and opening the envelope to read the contents, but then again it wasn't my business. I negated the idea.

Next was the blue folder, the wall safe. I found it easily behind an oil painting on the wall in the bedroom. The papers in the safe looked old, brittle, and yellow as if they hadn't been touched in many years. I carefully handled them and placed them in the blue folder. I was now half finished with the folders and had earned a break

I looked for and found the blanket I had used yesterday and curled up in front of the fireplace. It was hard to curl up with so many clothes on. In Phoenix I was used to shorts and sleeveless tops. Here I was in long sweats and a coat. It felt great though to sense coldness and winter in the air. I decided today was a good day to journal rather than read. I realized it has been many months since I had retired. I felt guilty because I didn't have and didn't want a job. I didn't even have a job description as a retiree and hadn't accomplished too much. Then I contradicted myself. I had completed the Master Gardener course, finished my watercolor picture, become a hiker, and a regular exerciser at the Club. Inside I felt so full knowing that each morning I could begin the day with a meditation. In the past my workday had often begun in anxiety.

Throughout my life I have read books and during the past several months of retirement I hadn't completed reading one book. The mind was a mystery. My favorite exploration in reading and experimenting with life was to discover how the mind worked. Not just any mind, but my mind. Look how quickly I had judged myself as inadequate because I didn't have a job. Much of my identity was tied up in my job for all those years. I knew I was a workaholic and maybe providing social services was my mission for that time period. The word mission had such religious overtones, but then again most businesses had mission statements. I thought of my friend Suzanne, and how I had supported her as she developed her personal mission statement. I made a mental note to pursue my personal mission statement. I had one but it was time for an update.

I looked at what I'd learned through the years and started jotting down notes. All of a sudden a zillion little thoughts bubbled up in my brain. I wrote as fast as I could until my paper was full. Some thoughts I forgot before I could write them. I rationalized; some thoughts were worth remembering and some weren't. My notes like thoughts are things; thought precedes form, create your day with your thoughts and feelings, sounded so trivial and yet was powerful. I knew I would never trade my hard earned knowledge for any amount of money. Not even for a million dollars. "No way," I said out loud, I love the little I knew about thinking and being in this world. I believed this life was a bridge and I do not begin or end here. Earth was a good place to learn and right now my only place to learn.

I savored these jobless moments of freedom. I knew I was free to be comfortable or scared. I had some scared thoughts about staying alone in the cabin. I wasn't sure of the root cause of my scared thoughts. I knew my thoughts created and if I was scared then I created something, anything, to frighten me. Thoughts created things. I decided to meditate on my oneness with all that was. I lit the candle from yesterday and sank into the pillows I had placed on the floor. The sound of the crackling fire was fading.

I focused on my breath, inhaling in peace and exhaling love. In the silence I sensed that fluidic intelligence as it flowed through every cell of my body. Peace encompassed me. I continued for about ten minutes and then opened my eyes. Everything always looked different to me when I came out of meditation. I could see and hear everything with clarity.

I sensed the fire needed some attention. Maybe more logs added would keep it going. I added logs. Thoughts of my spiritual teacher who had died several years ago surfaced. I felt so blessed and humbled by her example of living love. People always commented to me about my peacefulness, which I attributed to my teacher. I thanked them, but there was always a little piece of my psyche that said no, not me, my teacher yes, but not me. Yes, I wanted to be loving and supportive of all of me. I decided to journal with the part of myself that didn't think I deserved to be retired and peaceful.

Chapter 24

Who Goes There

A knock at the front door pierced my peace. I just about jumped up the chimney. I gathered my wits and laughed to myself. I heard someone knocking at the front door and yelling.

"Larry? Beth? Are you in there?" I looked through the upper window in the front door and saw an older couple with something in their hands. I opened the door and prayed for a peaceful encounter. The couple stared at me with a startled look. I introduced myself.

"Hi, I'm Nancy, Larry and Beth's neighbor in Phoenix."

Their faces relaxed.

"I'm Joe and this is my wife, Alice. We thought you were Larry and Beth. We brought over some homemade soup."

I motioned them in.

"Please come in, it's cold out there."

Joe extended his hands holding the soup and offered it to me.

"Here you enjoy the soup, Nancy."

I accepted and thanked them. They both took a seat on the couch and seemed very comfortable. I set the soup on the counter and settled in on the cushions on the floor. Alice was the first to speak.

"Late yesterday afternoon we thought we saw a red jeep pull out of the driveway. We were concerned and called Larry in Phoenix. He wasn't home so we left a message. We haven't heard back from him. We kind of were looking for the jeep today and thought Larry and Beth might be up here in a new car."

Joe pointed out the front window to a cabin down the road with smoke curling out of the chimney.

"That's where we live. We didn't see the jeep arrive today, but when we saw smoke from your chimney we decided to check it out. We can't see your car because it's parked in the back and not visible to us from our cabin. Larry probably didn't think we would still be up here in Strawberry. Actually we expected to be gone by now, but Alice is finishing some oil paintings of scenery in Strawberry for a show."

The two of them sat on the couch nestled in the big cushions that seemed to swallow them up. They would nod and grin first looking at one another and then at me. Alice kept her feet crossed at the anklebone and only shifted positions once. Joe was a jovial guy with rosy cheeks who fidgeted a lot. I sat on the floor and felt right at home with them and being in the cabin. Alice's gaze kept returning to the artwork on the walls. I could tell she enjoyed art.

"Anyway, we thought if you weren't Larry, you were one of the grandkids driving a red jeep. We were surprised to see anyone. Larry and Beth have both talked about their nice neighbor in Phoenix. I bet that nice neighbor is you."

"Thank you, many times they have invited me here, but I never made it. I see now what I missed and why they love Strawberry so much. Larry wanted me to stay here, but I was skeptical so I'm sleeping at the Strawberry Lodge."

"You could have stayed with us; we love it up here also." Joe smiled at Alice who nodded her head. It made me feel welcomed.

"I can't believe people call these cabins. When I think of cabin I envision a small one-room building. This is magnificent and the fireplace looks old and authentic with all the brickwork. Even the front door, I didn't expect it to open, it is just too pretty."

"Did Larry decide to sell this place? It wouldn't surprise me. He was having trouble caring for Beth in such a remote place. The nearest hospital is Payson, which is a twenty-mile drive from here. He was pretty sure the girls and grandkids weren't interested so he talked about putting it on the market from Phoenix."

"Gosh that I don't know."

All of sudden things made sense to me. No wonder the old papers looked as if no one had touched them for years, they hadn't. Maybe that was why he wanted his papers in Phoenix; he was getting ready to sell.

I updated them up on Beth's medical status and told them the name of the hospital.

"Nancy if you want heat in the cabin, let me know, I can work the propane tank. And I will turn it off for you after you leave."

"Thanks Joe that sounds great, it you don't mind, I would appreciate some heat." Joe went outside and made some adjustments to the tank.

"I am staying at the Strawberry Lodge in town, but tonight, especially since I have heat, I may just stay the night. I am smitten by this cabin. It would be a treat for a city girl."

Alice smiled. She knew the beauty of Strawberry. When Joe came back in Alice looked up at him.

"We need to move along." And then she looked at me. "We're glad everything is okay." She took a pencil from her purse, wrote down their phone number, and handed it to me.

"Nancy call us if you need anything and let us know when you leave. Why don't you come to our house for breakfast? We usually eat around eight. Whether you decide to stay all night or drive back to the lodge come and eat breakfast with us."

Joe reiterated the invitation, which made me feel doubly welcomed. "Even if you go back to the hotel come early for pancakes. Alice makes great pancakes."

Joe and Alice left through the front door. It made me feel powerful to actually shut the mammoth front door.

Chapter 25

A Little Heat Goes a Long Way

I felt the heat from the propane tank kick in. The soup on the counter was still warm to the touch. It was time for lunch. I found a spoon in the drawer and washed if off. The aroma of the soup filled my senses. It was chicken noodle with big pieces of carrot. It was enough for two people. I dug in.

In my heart I believed everything was sacred; now if I saw it and realized it all the time I would be in heaven. Yes it was easy to feel loving and compassionate toward kind and loving people like Joe and Alice. The rub for me was to feel love and compassion toward the people I didn't like. Maybe it wasn't the people, but rather what the people were doing that I didn't like. Give it a rest I thought. Just enjoy the soup. I discovered more vegetables floating in the rich broth. This was heaven in front of a fireplace. I gave thanks for the unexpected treat. I felt nurtured.

It was near three pm, my planned time to let the fire die and head back to the lodge. It was decision time. Either I prepared to leave or stay the night. It was easy and I placed some more wood on the fire. I called the Strawberry Lodge just to let them know I would not be returning that evening, but would return the following evening.

"I don't want anyone to think I skipped out."

"Thank you for being considerate."

I sat and rested on the couch for a few minutes. My mind floated back to Denny's and I thought about my new intention that I had composed to being loving and supportive. What began as an Annie thing evolved into a respect for setting intention. The repetition of that intention, to be loving and supportive, kept the wheels of my brain turning. Without doubt I knew my meditation had set the tone for my day. When thoughts of fear crept into my mind, like being alone in the cabin, I reminded myself to trust and pray. The Intelligence, the God that created the planets in the universe was certainly guiding me in this tiny town of Strawberry. My spiritual teacher had taught me to wash my hands of fear, to watch the fear circle and go down the sink. And then she had instructed me to replace the fear thoughts with trust, joy and love. Remembering that teaching, I immediately went into the bathroom and washed my hands.

It was time, I thought, to return to my folder status. The first three folders were completed. The second and third folders, green and blue, contained their respective papers. Old and crumpled the title and personal papers were accounted for. The book and wall safe were empty. The fourth folder was white and I hadn't started it yet.

I picked it up and followed the map to the shed. I unlocked and opened the door of the shed. I retrieved the weed eater that Larry had requested be returned to Phoenix. I also noted again the red arrow printed on his directions that pointed to a shovel. I wasn't sure what the shovel was for, but I picked it up and carried it along with the weed eater to my car. Out of the corner of my eye in the far distance I could make out the silhouette of a man walking his dog. I bet it was the same man I'd seen in the cowboy hat with his dog. No point in waving to him, he was too far away. Weed eater and shovel were checked off my list of to dos in the white folder. I returned to the shed and locked the door. I returned to the house.

It felt cozy to enter a warm cabin. The white folder went back in the box and I considered it completed. I reached for the fifth folder. It was red and included a map with directions to a space behind the shed. The directions indicated digging in this space behind the shed; I was to dig for a box.

"Wow, me digging, no way."

The ground was hard and almost frozen. I reread the directions. This time I focused on the word in the corner, optional. Larry had printed "optional" in parenthesis. I must have missed it in my first read. Knowing me I may have tried it the following day, but the optional gave me a way out. It was too cold and the ground too hard.

In my mind I tried to remember why I had thought I had a key to the basement in one of these folders. Maybe I thought it was basement because Larry referred to the depth of digging as basement level. There was a key, but I concluded it was to open whatever was found in the dig. What I did know was I had to read carefully. I was aware of the power of words and this one word, basement, I had misunderstood. I was human and my intention to be loving and supportive took over.

Chapter 26

One Folder Left

Ahh, one folder left and it was bright yellow. When I finished this one I could truly relax for the evening. I checked the woodpile next to the fireplace. It appeared to be plenty, but my instinct guided me to bring more inside. Outside I went and it was colder. I picked up wood and examined it for bugs. It was too cold for bugs I told myself. The cabin was getting dirtier each time I entered, but the cabin could be cleaned easily enough. Livable, not perfect, was the way I would describe my house.

I still had granola bars and if I got real hungry I could help myself to the freezer food. I wasn't sure if the freezer was working. The phone worked, but I didn't know how. I embarrassed myself by being ignorant of how these utilities functioned. The electricity worked just fine. It had to be just the heat that was on the propane tank. It made me question how many things in life I had missed because I didn't understand the basics. A person can't see or hold a piece of electricity in their hand yet the effects of electricity are demonstrated by turning on a light switch. It was a rationale I used to explain the Presence of God. Any use of definition by virtue of defining included and excluded concepts. God was and is everything. Everything from the purest snow to the sludge in the sewer was an effect of God. All was included and none was excluded. In my mind no one could come up with any place or thing where God was not.

I glanced out the window and noticed snowflakes falling, some sticking on the glass pane. It was mystical and a perfect way to open the last folder. I carefully read the directions; "under the rug is a loose board." The ink on the paper from the final yellow folder was smudged. It wasn't clear. The rug Larry referenced was definitely the living room rug. There was an asterisk on the directions and it was as small as the fine print in a contract. The asterisk stated, "contents to be either destroyed or given to Larry and only to Larry." Larry was underlined. How strange I thought, but whatever Larry wanted was okay by me. Anyway I would prefer looking for a loose floorboard rather than digging in frozen earth.

I added several logs to the fire and began looking for the loose floorboard. I rolled back the rug and ran my hands over the wood floor. Within ten minutes I felt one of the boards move to my touch. Gingerly I pried and lifted the board up. My heart danced as my eyes viewed an old burlap bag poking out from a tin box underneath the floorboard. How cool! With both hands I raised the bag up out of the earth. Inside the bag was a yellowing manuscript along with some old newspaper clippings. I was afraid to touch the paper for fear they would crumble in my hands. Carefully I placed the manuscript with newspaper clippings on the dining table. I returned to the loose board and made sure I had removed all of the contents from the cavity under the floor. It was dark outside now and, just to be sure, I checked all the windows and doors to make certain they were locked. It was going to be a long night.

I replaced the rug over the loose board and felt like I solved a mystery. A cup of tea sounded great so I headed for the kitchen. The stove was electric and I placed a kettle of water on to boil. Rummaging through other people's cupboards seemed strange. It was worth my rummage however, because my hand rested on a box of Earl Grey tea. Earl Grey tea and granola bars went well together. The manuscript was on the table and seemed to have a magnet that drew me to it. It felt as if I would be invading Larry's privacy if I looked at the contents. It was none of my business and Larry had specifically directed that it be returned to him and only to him or be destroyed. Yes, I knew that meant for his eyes only but…but…there was always a "but." But preceded what a person really wanted to say. Before the word "but" were couch words to lighten or ease into the real message. But, I wanted to read the manuscript. I could rationalize anything. Usually I used my powers of rationalization to purchase things I didn't really need. Larry's envelope and personal papers I understood to be personal, but a manuscript hidden in such an inconspicuous place enticed me. Then there was the buried box by the shed. In my mind I bargained to dig it up tomorrow no matter what in exchange for reading the document. I could soak the area with water and dig tomorrow. It was easier to dig after being soaked, but with the snow it would freeze. I negated both ideas again.

The stars outside began glistening through the upper glass windowpanes over the front door. I could see stars and a piece of the moon among the snow flurries. Snow was so pure. It was white and white supposedly represented purity, but what if snow was orange or brown? My psyche would have a strong reaction if it were other than white. White was like a blank piece of paper that could contain anything at all. The first pencil mark on any white sheet of paper could be seen like snow angels in the snow. White represented the blank, the nothingness or all potential. Pure black maybe did the same but black, like at night, can't be seen. What can't be seen is more frightening because it was unknown. The lightness or brightness of white doesn't do that. Out of the unknown or darkness creativity was born.

Color was so important. There was color in racism. All I knew for sure was that all races were red inside because all of our blood was red. White people, like me, weren't really white. We were this pinky beige and we always looked better with a suntan. Yet there were whites who disliked darker skinned people and there were dark skinned people who disliked light skinned people. The wars over God and the wars over race were so dysfunctional. I thought about all the times in my life when I was dysfunctional, even before I knew the word existed and what it meant. There were many people I needed to apologize to for my ignorance. And many who owed that service to me. I thought about the term the great white brotherhood and the KKK. I wondered if there were a great black brotherhood based on spirituality or maybe they were the black masons. Every culture or race must have something like shamans, medicine men, elders of the race. There was always someone who risked going out there in the realm of the unknown only to return with pearls of great price. I had heard of hundreds of them and maybe even met one or two.

Except for the slight sound of the crackling fire the silence in the room was deafening. The smell of cedar wood burning permeated the air. I was so alone, so vulnerable. Here I was a city girl alone in the middle of who knows where on a cold night with the closest other human several blocks away in a cabin. I learned about telling the truth and not fooling myself. Okay, okay, the truth was in that moment I was afraid of my aloneness and vulnerability. I embraced my fear. At home I had a burglar alarm system that shrieked and signaled the police if a break-in occurred. It would take a long time for police to get to Strawberry. I noticed a fire, but no police station on my drive through town. My guess was the police were stationed in Payson. I tried to and couldn't remember the name of the people across the street who had brought me the soup. My mind drew a blank. I took some deep breaths and focused in the present moment. Oh yes the neighbors' names were Joe and Alice. I looked at my watch and it was now almost eight pm.

I decided to call Joe and Alice under the guise of accepting their invitation for breakfast. Oh yes and by the way I would ask them what number to call in case of an emergency. My call was quick and priceless. Joe was my contact.

"I'm glad you called Nancy and we are thrilled you will join us for breakfast. We like entertaining city slickers like you."

"Hey Joe, what does a person up here do in case of an emergency?"

"You hit redial on the phone and I'll be over with my gun. Not to worry, if you get scared I'll drive over, pick you up, and you can spend the night with us. It doesn't matter what time it is just call us. There is always 911 for emergency, but you know that."

"Thanks Joe."

My voice sounded relieved. It was good to know 911 was up here.

The fear of being alone was deeper than the physical and maybe had nothing at all to do with the physical. I rationalized; I came into the world alone and will leave alone. There were people all around me at my birth because I was born in a hospital. Yet my first breath the actual realization of being human was an alone journey. I'd been re-birthed several times. I recalled several rebirthings one in particular was in the water, in a pool. The accentuated breath under the direction of a trained facilitator took many of us back in memory to birth. Some went back in time for healing and some for experience. I decided it was a good time in that moment for me to meditate and trust in my own being, just like at birth. After all, my own being was still alive and healthy at age fifty-seven.

It amazed me how loud a room could be when it was filled with just my breath. I listened to the rhythm of my inhale and exhale. My gut quieted in the stillness and all my senses were enhanced. In that moment absolutely nothing was missing in my life. It was as though my body emanated a light, the essence of peace. In my mind I was like a snowflake floating in the universe with this sense of being all important when in reality I'm was just a little snowflake. Yet even the snowflake was a piece of the universe and all that was. That which created the snowflake was God, the all that was and is. Big and small we all were important.

A snowflake experienced the freedom of falling, of being. Humans had awareness and free will. A falling snowflake taught me the mystery of freedom. The snowflake was free to be a snowflake. No choices and no awareness. Humans had choices and a possible choice was to pretend to be someone other than self.

My spiritual mentor taught me that a person who truly meditated could meditate in Times Square and not be affected. A snowflake could fall in Times Square or here in Arizona and still be a snowflake. The experience of being a snowflake was not dependent on location. My mentor finished that lesson and added, but only a damn fool would meditate in Times Square. I sensed all of the unity in my life, all the emotions, feelings and thoughts. I expressed freedom every day, every moment of my life only now I expressed with conscious awareness. Now I was like an aware snowflake; aware of being and aware of the choice to be aware. The mystery of freedom implied choice, free will; it had to. I prayed for continuing wisdom and a peaceful night's sleep and, of course, if any of my dreams needed to be remembered it would happen easily, lovingly, and gently. I ended my prayer time in gratitude, a true grace.

Chapter 27

Sleeping in the Cabin

My pajamas were back in the motel. I didn't relish the idea of sleeping in clothes that I planned on wearing the next day. I rummaged in Larry and Beth's bedroom and came up with a flannel nightgown that must have belonged to Beth. I could launder it at home and return it to Larry in Phoenix. After all I knew I was going to glance at that manuscript that I dug up from under the floorboards. In Beth's gown I felt more a part of the family.

I was glad I had retrieved additional logs outside and brought them into the house. It was possibly going to turn into an all nighter. I had nowhere to go tomorrow other than breakfast with Joe and Alice. Even my return to the Strawberry Lodge was optional. With extra logs the fire roared as I moved toward the dining room table. I gently lifted the manuscript leaving the old newspaper clippings flat down on the table. I headed for the cushion by the fire, curled into the blanket, and untied the brittle rope from around the old manuscript. I estimated that the manuscript was about fifty pages in length. I would remember to suggest to Larry that he let me type it on my computer. It would be easy to make copies. I knew if I made that suggestion, I would have to admit I had read his manuscript. I was okay with that. It was the truth. No excuses, I was excited to start reading.

Before I could start the phone in the cabin rang. It was Alice.

"Nancy, Joe can pick you up and you can sleep over here. We have plenty of room. You might be afraid over there by yourself."

"No thanks, Alice I've never felt better and safer."

It was the truth.

"We're off to sleep then, we will see you for pancakes."

"Oh that sounds great Alice, would you mind making sure I am awake, maybe around seven or seven-fifteen? Just to make sure I am awake."

"No problem."

We said our goodnights.

I returned to my place in front of the fire and focused on the manuscript. The first couple pages of the manuscript were blank. Then there was the title page in big hand written letters, "THE MAN AND HIS DOG." The next page in smaller hand printed letters read "Chapter 1 — The Frontiers of Arizona"...and so the story began, at least for me the reader.

To my amazement the whole manuscript was written by hand. I knew this had to be old. I was extremely careful in turning pages, desperate not to let them tear. I reminded myself again to ask Larry if he wanted me to type it on my computer for posterity. I knew I would have to wait to see Larry's reaction to me reading it. Larry's directions had been clear; "either it is to be destroyed or given to me (Larry) and only to him (Larry)." I was violating his request, but I was just reading it and not keeping it. I snuggled deeper in the blanket and started the first chapter.

The story began around 1900 as told to the author of the manuscript. I assumed the author was Larry. No author was listed on the title page. Arizona being the old Wild West had plenty of mines, copper and otherwise. Unions were popping up all over the country and Arizona was no exception. The manuscript story began in Jerome, Arizona in July of 1900. Jerome was an old copper mining town. A group of mine workers approached the "Western Federation of Miners" and requested a charter. It was granted. A week later five hundred member signed up for the union. As with any union they had rights, which included strikes for better pay and working conditions. It was rumored that if management got wind of strikes the mines would close for repair. Management figured if the miners got hungry enough they would return to work no matter the conditions. As a result most strikes were not successful. Mines would reopen and the miners return to the same or worse conditions. It was very convenient for the mine owners.

Arizona became a state in 1912. The political climate supported unions. The "Western Federation of Miners" was succeeded by the "The International Union of Mine, Mill, and Smelter Workers" (IUMMSW). A second smaller union to protect about five hundred Mexican workers was called the "Ligi Protectora Latina." And a third union was called the "International Workers of the World Union" (IWW). The unions lacked communication and common goals as were printed in the story because the unions competed for membership. The IWW was the most aggressive, and proactive in their demands for change. Management considered them out of line for making unjustified demands.

World War I became a reality. The miners in Jerome were more concerned about survival than serving in the military. Many miners were of European descent and a large percentage was German. Miners from Mexico certainly had a need to unionize under the Ligi Protectora Latina Union. Miners, as described and told to the author of this manuscript, were hard working and from every possible ethnic group. Their workdays were long and little, if any, medical care was provided. Accidents were normal in mines. These Jerome miners were not allowed to move families with them to Jerome. Boarding houses populated Jerome. Naturally the bordellos followed. How awful to not allow the families and then allow bordellos. It made me think this is how administration controlled the miners. Once when I was in Alaska I visited a mine that had been set up as its own community. That place had a different feel about it with cottages and a school for the miner's children. The miners in Jerome were treated like indentured slaves. Without their families booze and bordellos tempted them.

Management and the unions distrusted each other. Distrust between and among the three unions complicated things even more. Most of the negative publicity for unions was because of the IWW nicknamed the Wobblies. The Wobblies believed in bum work if they didn't receive good pay. The Wobblies rose to fame because they threatened to harm anyone and everyone who got in their way. Many Arizonians considered the threatening behavior of the Wobblies as un-American. Hysteria began. The author of this manuscript made it clear that the Wobblies were active in Kingman and Bisbee mines as well. I was shocked that I could live in Arizona this many years and not have realized this history. Then again I had never read any history books on Arizona. Maybe it wasn't even a true story I was reading in the manuscript. Larry would tell me.

Chapter 28

The Manuscript Continues

Chapter two of the manuscript was titled "Patrick." Patrick with no last name was a miner of Irish descent who wanted to work and help his family back in Ireland immigrate to America. Patrick was born on February twentieth, eighteen ninety-eight. He was big, tall, and strong. Although he was intellectually smart he was politically naïve. His Uncle Bill paid for him to get to America for a new start. Uncle Bill was an older gregarious hard working and hard drinking Irishman nicknamed Chubby. Chubby was a popular cartoon character and the nickname stuck. Even Patrick called his Uncle Bill by the nickname of Chubby. They landed in New York after a strenuous ship ride from Ireland. They worked on the rail lines through the Appalachian Mountains. Neither of them was afraid of hard labor and both desired to keep their noses out of politics, which was unusual for Irishmen. Both worked in the coalmines of Appalachia for extremely long hours and low pay. They celebrated being in America. Neither Patrick nor Chubby belonged to a union.

One day Chubby was killed in a terrible mine accident, an accident that easily could have been prevented. Patrick was heartbroken and considered it murder. Patrick was afraid that management would come after him to keep him quiet about the conditions surrounding Chubby's death. Patrick knew the circumstances and felt it was plain old murder. Before the murder/accident Patrick and Chubby had planned to move out west and earn their fortunes together as a team. Patrick, in all his sorrow, decided it was best for him to continue with the plan even if he was without his beloved Chubby. Patrick felt his life was in danger if he stayed. He decided to go west. He knew he could best honor Chubby's memory by becoming successful. He promised himself to return to Appalachia one day and place a beautiful headstone on Chubby's grave. For right now Patrick needed all his money for the move. There wasn't much money left after he paid for Chubby's burial expenses and, of course, some good ole Irish whiskey to drown his sorrows. Irish whiskey was mandatory for an Irish wake. Patrick in all his grief managed to make his way to Arizona.

Chapter three in the manuscript was titled "Patrick in Jerome." It was early in April according to the manuscript when Patrick reached Arizona. As best as he could, Patrick worked his way across the country from Appalachia to Arizona via Roman Catholic Churches. Catholic churches had always welcomed the Irish Catholic Americans. Although Patrick didn't consider himself involved in politics he knew that being an Irish Catholic in America was synonymous with voting the democratic ticket. The Roman Catholic Churches across the country provided him with safe job leads and meals, which many times were meager, but a meal none the less. This part of the manuscript rang true to me. My distant Irish roots included women running boarding homes for teamsters. It sounded feasible to me and typical of early immigrants. They took care of their own as best as they could. I could accept this network as true.

Once in Arizona Patrick was given several leads for job openings for miners in Kingman, Bisbee and Jerome. He was told his best bet was Jerome. It was impossible to properly explain the heat of Arizona to a non-desert dweller from Ireland. Drink water became his mantra. Prior to his arrival in Jerome Patrick was handed a paper with a contact name, Al. There was no last name. He was told he could find Al at the House of Joy in Jerome. Al would advise and guide him.

It took Patrick several hours by train to reach Jerome. Jerome sat high on the side of a hill surrounded by a thick dense forest. Any way into the town was rocky with narrow paths, similar to Appalachia. Only Appalachia was cooler and not so dusty.

Patrick noticed the red veins running through all the rocks and called them rock embers. He found Jerome extremely beautiful and extremely hot.

He came upon the House of Joy and to his shock it was a bordello. That day in Jerome must have been a payday because the House of Joy was hopping. People were on the porches and a crowd was partying in the street in front of the building. Patrick couldn't quite connect getting a referral to a bordello from a Catholic Church acquaintance. Here Patrick was in the middle of it all and everyone was liquored up. Patrick had seen drinking of this type more times than he cared to remember. He felt trapped.

He made his way to what had to be the front door and asked for the name on his piece of paper, Al. A friendly face in the crowd responded to Patrick and ushered him to the rear of the building. A small man with spectacles appeared. They met. Patrick read deep sorrow in Al's eyes that reminded him of his own sorrow about Uncle Bill, Chubby.

The two men, Al and Patrick talked. It became apparent to Patrick that Al was not the typical miner. Patrick learned that Al was a go between for management who expected Al to thwart any attempts at union formation. It wasn't working well for management because, as Al told it to Patrick, there were currently three unions in Jerome.

AL took an immediate liking to Patrick and decided that he would take Patrick under his wing. Privately, Al knew Patrick was alone and needed guidance especially without his Uncle Bill. Al had met other young men similar to Patrick, but they didn't have the stamina and genuineness of Patrick. Al hoped Patrick would remain that way, but he had his doubts. Jerome was very political, with management disrespect and miner unrest.

Al had thought of leaving Jerome because he couldn't stand living there without his family. No one other than management was permitted to live with his family in Jerome. Management thought that family would interfere with work. Management could get more work out of the miners if their families weren't around or so they believed. Management had concerns around the possibility of wives, women organizing for the rights of their husbands. After all the women would have time with their husbands working long shifts. Any talk of union was not greeted well by administration and any man who favored unions became a marked man.

As I read I could see in my mind's eye some of the places that the author referenced so many years ago. The "House of Joy" became a restaurant I had frequented back in the eighties. In the manuscript The House of Joy was a brothel where the overworked and underpaid men found solace. It was anything but joyous according to this story. The author heard all this from a man named Patrick with no last name. I finished the chapter and made a cup of decaffeinated tea all the time thinking about Jerome.

In the manuscript the mine hired Patrick. He was excited to start work. Al had helped Patrick find a boarding house room. Patrick felt as if he was starting his new life.

Chapter 29

More about Patrick

Patrick completed his first full month as a miner in Jerome. Things began to heat up inside the unions and management disregarded any requests for better working conditions. There was a lot of rock throwing and demands. The Wobblies were in high gear. In spite of it all Patrick, the miner, and AL, pseudo management guy, shared Sunday dinners. AL confided many, many things to Patrick. Al knew Patrick was a solid young man. Al was quite glad that Patrick hadn't joined a union, which would have ended their friendship, at least in public.

One of the confidences Al shared and bragged about with Patrick was a little piece of land he had purchased in Strawberry, Arizona. Al was proud to own the land. His dream was to move his wife and their two children to Strawberry and farm the land. Al was sick of management and the unions. He understood the plight of the miner and the abuse many of them had experienced at the hands of management. He also knew in the final analysis the miner didn't stand a chance against management.

Patrick disagreed because he thought there was always hope and everyone stood a chance if they trusted in life, and trusted in God. Patrick tried unsuccessfully to encourage Al to trust. Patrick was a Catholic, no doubt. Al and Patrick respected and trusted each other.

Because of that trust one day Al arranged for Patrick to deliver some papers for him to Prescott, Arizona. Al explained the privacy of the papers and that no one, including Patrick, was to read them. Al paid Patrick handsomely. Al, himself, could not leave Jerome. Management would not hear of it. There were too many management issues going on. In fact, management had called an emergency meeting for July 9, 1917, at the Jerome High School. Al was mandated to attend.

Chapter 30

Welcome to Prescott

I got sleepy and began to doze. I didn't want to fall asleep while reading such a fragile document. I could accidentally damage it. I was close to finishing it and I couldn't stop. I got up, sat in an upright chair and ate another granola bar. This document was too cool. I didn't know and didn't care what time it was. I wanted to finish. I placed my attention back on the manuscript. I read on.

Patrick made his way to the stagecoach for the trip to Prescott. Al had talked to him the night before and given him all the instructions. According to Al's instructions Patrick was to spend one night in Prescott and return the next day to Jerome. Patrick had few possessions and didn't have much to pack for a one-day trip. It was the first time Patrick had spent the night in a boarding house paid for by someone else. It seemed like a waste of money to him because his bed in Jerome was paid for and empty.

Al had arranged for Patrick to spend the night with a friend in Prescott. Patrick was used to being directed to people he didn't know. He met many people including Al through referrals. It made Patrick wonder what he ever would have done had he not been given all the names of people he had met all along his journey to Arizona. Patrick boarded the coach with papers and a bag in hand.

I breezed through the chapter describing the scenery that Patrick was seeing on his way to Prescott. I was familiar with the beauty. Plus I knew I could re-read that section tomorrow, but for now I wanted to finish the manuscript.

Patrick arrived on schedule in Prescott on July ninth. He recalled that Al's emergency meeting at the high school would take place that evening. He wasn't sure of the start time but he thought it was around six pm. He hoped Al would have a good meeting. Patrick had wished for Al to trust more in life. Patrick took comfort in knowing that he was taking care of business for Al in Prescott. Maybe Al would trust more as a result of Patrick. He was glad to have Al as a friend. Patrick questioned why AL didn't just wait until after the emergency meeting and go to Prescott himself. Patrick rationalized that Al was just too busy and probably not allowed by management to ever leave Jerome.

Patrick arrived at the boarding house where Al had arranged for him to spend the night. The proprietor of the boarding house was a long time friend of Al's. Patrick took to him immediately. The proprietor gave Patrick a map to the location where he was to meet another man very early the next morning and deliver Al's papers. The proprietor invited Patrick to dine with him that evening because, after all, Patrick was a friend of Al's.

Chapter 31

The Meeting

Patrick arrived at the arranged meeting location fifteen minutes early. He liked the ruggedness of Prescott. It was the capitol for Arizona and it was a hub of activity with lots of animals especially horses all around. When it was time for his meeting, another man appeared and to Patrick's surprise the other man was the proprietor. He was meeting with the proprietor of the boarding house where he had stayed last night and who he had dinner with last evening. In fact their plan was to meet up for coffee before Patrick returned to Jerome. The proprietor was formal and asked Patrick for the sealed envelop with Al's papers.

The proprietor continued the meeting. He looked Patrick in the eye.

"You are a very lucky man Patrick. What you don't know Patrick is that Al has arranged for you to start a new life. I am sure that you are aware of the union dangers brewing in Jerome. People across the country are panicked by the IWW threats to do physical harm if the IWW demands are not met. Management and the people are very upset, as I am sure you know. In the short time that you have known Al you have impressed him with all your talk about trusting life. In every letter I have received from him he has talked about your faith. He was in complete awe of your trusting faith in the middle of this chaos."

Patrick was in shock at the complimentary words.

"As you probably will hear in the next day or two things are very different in Jerome than when you left yesterday. It is a very dangerous place right now for the miners. Al does not want you to return to Jerome at all, ever. There is talk of deporting miners for their disobedience to management. Al himself is on his way out of town. He left during the night and is heading back east to be with his wife and children. His wife will not under any circumstance live anywhere in or near Arizona. Al had mentioned to you he has a piece of property in Strawberry. It isn't worth much money, but he wants you to have it. If anything ever happens to Al he might show up in Strawberry, but he doubts it. His wife, back east, just inherited some money. Al doesn't plan on ever leaving the East again. The condition of his gift of land to you is that you never disclose the source of the gift. I am prepared to put your name on the document and register the title at the capitol on that condition. What do you think?"

Patrick, according to the author's source, was speechless. A million thoughts ran through his mind.

"What danger? What land? Where is Strawberry Arizona? Of course I would never tell."

Patrick wiped sweat and a tear from his eye. Inside his heart broke. It was another loss of a friend, this time Al. First he lost Chubby and now his friend AL. In Patrick's mind, according to the author's source, the word trust surfaced. Patrick signed the paperwork.

The proprietor explained that Patrick's room in Prescott was paid up for the week compliments of Al. The suggestion was made that it would be wiser for Patrick to leave by the end of the week. The proprietor looked sad.

"Something bad is happening in Jerome. Inside this envelope is your cash from your final wages in Jerome, Al had thought of everything."

Patrick looked overwhelmed. The proprietor gave him a comforting look.

"Maybe at dinner tonight you can share your thoughts on trust with me. It is best for everyone if you do not try to contact Al at all. You understand? With all of the unrest in Jerome it is best that neither one of you try to communicate. However there may be a day when Al shows up in Strawberry. Al's last words to you are "thank you for teaching me about trust. May we both be happy and trust in life, in God. God bless you."

I flipped through the manuscript to the chapter titled "Jerome Deportation." I didn't believe such a thing could really happen in the USA.

According to the author of the manuscript Patrick had overheard an official telling others about what happened in Jerome on July tenth, the day after the meeting and the same day Patrick found out he was getting the land in Strawberry. In the wee morning hours of July tenth, nineteen hundred and seventeen, vigilantes went to the boarding houses of Jerome and rounded up all possible members of the IWW or Wobblies. The Wobblies were accused of rock throwing, fistfights, and threats. At gunpoint they were put in cattle cars headed for Needles, California. Along the way the train was met by posses to make sure the Wobblies didn't get off. It was rumored that two or more Wobblies were added to the cattle car along the way. When the cattle car reached Needles, California the cattle car was rejected by California and eventually the Wobblies were freed. The Wobblies promised never to agitate again. They were released into the desert. And that was the end of the Wobblies.

Chapter 32

The Last Chapter of the Manuscript

The last chapter of the manuscript was titled "Strawberry." According to the manuscript Patrick eventually made it to Strawberry. Along the way he followed his routine and contacted churches and names the proprietor had given him. Patrick found his little piece of land and was mesmerized by the beauty and diversity. There was even a stray dog that wondered the land. Patrick adopted the dog and named him Trust.

According to the manuscript Patrick gave some information about his marriage and children who came along several years after he had arrived in Strawberry. He emphasized to the author of the manuscript that the story was about a man, a little piece of paper, trust, and a dog named Trust. Patrick never let go of the little piece of paper that listed his name, Patrick, on the deed as the rightful owner. The first time Patrick discussed it with any one was with the author of this manuscript in my hand. The only reason Patrick shared the information with the author was because Patrick was getting ready to transfer the land to his son-in-law. The transfer, in the spirit of Al, was to be in the strictness of confidence. All I could think about was the thoughtfulness of Al. Given the same circumstances I doubted I would be so kind. People today don't just give away property, well, at least that I've heard about. Al fit in with the spirit of the old Wild West and certainly with Arizona history. There weren't a lot of homegrown Arizonians during that time. People came out west to discover gold, to build, to get away. Whatever their reasons they had to be tough and strong to endure. I picked up the manuscript.

Oh yes, Patrick told the author, the proprietor in Prescott who was so kind to him so many years ago went on to become the Mayor of Prescott. It seemed that no one ever discovered how Patrick came about his land. Everyone knew about Patrick's trust in life and, of course, his dog named Trust. Even though Patrick was dead, on some days it was said that a person could see the old man, Patrick, and his dog, Trust, walking along the outskirts of Strawberry as a reminder for everyone to trust.

Chapter 33

Return to Now

Feeling dazed I closed the manuscript and placed it back on the dining room table. I returned to the couch, sat, and was silent for a long time. It was after one AM and I was exhausted. I stretched out on the couch, pulled the extra blankets over me, and fell fast asleep. The next thing I knew the phone was ringing. God only knew how long I would have slept had the phone not awakened me.

I dragged myself to the phone on the tenth ring. It was Alice.

"Good morning Nancy, this is your wake up call. It is seven fifteen and coffee is waiting for you."

"Thanks Alice I'll be there in a half hour or so, I just rolled out of bed. Is that okay?"

"Take your time Nancy, we're just relaxing. We're retired you know."

I figured out the shower and freshened up in the guest bathroom. Yesterday's clothes felt yucky next to my clean skin. Maybe if I pretended they were fresh from the dryer I would feel better. It worked. I have a good imagination.

I re-entered the living room, which looked bare without a roaring fire in the fireplace. My eye caught the manuscript and I smiled. I had lots of questions for Joe and Alice, but I couldn't be too direct otherwise I would have to tell them about the manuscript I wasn't supposed to have read. It was Shakespeare I thought who said something like "oh what a tangled web we weave when we at first start to deceive." I placed a cushion on the floor, sat on it, and spent fifteen minutes in meditation. I contemplated the wisdom that lived in my being.

It was time to go for pancakes. I opened the front door and felt as if I was leaving a cocoon. It was definitely cold outside; way colder than Phoenix and there was a fresh layer of snow maybe an inch of it. I locked the cabin door and headed for Joe and Alice's cabin in my jeep. Usually I brought some kind of a little thank you gift when I was invited for a meal, but I had nothing but granola bars. I pulled up behind their SUV and immediately heard a dog inside barking.

The sound of a barking dog invoked a deep sense of peace for me. I was thinking about Patrick and his dog, Trust. I reached the front door and all three of us converged on one another simultaneously. It was funny. Even their dog, Cutie, got in the act; the dog was insistent I pet him and I did. The smell of coffee greeted my nostrils and it was strong smelling coffee. Starbucks coffee had nothing on Joe and Alice. Alice held out a cup of black coffee to me and I accepted.

"Ahh yes coffee please."

Their kitchen was full of memorabilia and looked like a photo out of a county living magazine. There were pictures of children and grandchildren. There were oil paintings of trees, of mountains, of running water and open space. I made a comment.

"I feel like your kitchen is hugging me, it is so warm in color."

It was also warm temperature wise, but the colors made me feel right at home almost as if I had been here many times.

"You know Joe and Alice; this kitchen reflects your warm hearts." I ran my fingers over the blue gingham place mats and napkins. In the window was a yellow ceramic duck with a matching blue gingham apron. Alice patted my hand.

"It has taken us many years to make the cabin comfortable and homey. Now we are at home here in Strawberry."

Joe volunteered to give me a brief tour while Alice made the blueberry pancakes. Joe and I entered their living room with a large fireplace that was equal in beauty to Larry and Beth's fireplace. I stood in awe.

"To this Phoenix gal this big glowing fireplace is a work of art, you know that?"

"Yes, we know. It's a shame Larry's kids and grandkids hardly ever use the cabin, it is in such a beautiful spot."

"I'm sure that you know this but one of his daughters lives in Germany and the other in New Mexico?"

"I do, and it was terrible when that oldest girl was killed. Maybe the grandkids will get the bug to visit here. It has been years since any of the family other than Larry and Beth has been up here." Joe motioned me toward the hallway.

"We can sit in the living room in front of the fire after breakfast, and have a second or third cup of coffee." We moved down the hall.

"Sounds like a plan to me." I clutched my coffee in my hands. Joe pointed to the master bedroom.

"The floor is solid wood; the fireplace is small but nice for a bedroom this size and look at that large picture window. Through the years we've had many an animal peep through that window, the animals always look startled if they see us. We see them eye to eye, it's pretty great." On the bed I noticed the most beautiful handmade quilt.

"That quilt is beautiful."

"It's very, very, old, handed down from Alice's mother and originally from Amish country, Indiana, I think." The artwork on the wall was woodsy, vibrant in color, and congruent with the area.

"It is mostly Alice's work." Joe informed me. The master bathroom adjoined their bedroom and it had all the conveniences of home. Next on my tour was the guest room.

"This guest room is larger than my bedroom back in Phoenix. The paintings throughout your house are breathtaking. And the quilts on both beds are elegant. It contributes to the tranquility of your home. Would the two of you come and do this for my house?"

"I gotta tell Alice that one." Joe guided me past the last room in the back of the cabin.

"This is Alice's art studio and you can see this piece here is just about finished, this is the piece we were telling you about last night. We've stayed in Strawberry, past our expected departure date, so Alice could finish this piece for the Strawberry Chamber of Commerce fundraiser. As soon as she finishes it we are out of here. We'll be heading for our other home, probably in the next couple of days. Will you be up here longer than that?"

"Oh no Joe, I may be leaving as early as this afternoon."

A look of relief came over Joe's face.

"Good because I want to be here to disconnect your propane tank when you leave. And don't forget to remind Larry to call the Strawberry Electric Company to shut off his electricity in the cabin for the rest of the winter. I'm sure in Larry's hurry to get Beth back to Phoenix he forgot."

We both heard Alice call us to the kitchen for breakfast.

"Come and get em." Alice yelled with a sparkle in her voice.

"They smell like pancakes from heaven to me." I beat Joe to the kitchen.

Chapter 34

Breakfast

The three of us enjoyed one another's company. We laughed a lot as we got to know one another. After I gracefully devoured three large pancakes we moved into the living room for that second cup of coffee. Mine was actually a third cup. I had some questions.

"Who is that elderly gentleman with the cowboy hat? I've seen him several times walking with a big dog. Usually I've seen him near the turnoff after the Old School House."

Joe and Alice looked at their dog, Cutie. Cutie was a small cocker spaniel and about half the size of the dog I had seen walking with the elderly gentleman. I had barely asked my question when Joe and Alice began howling in laughter. I was puzzled and confused by their laughter.

"Did Larry put you up to this?"

I shook my head no.

"It's been years. Larry and I used to tease each other about some ghost guy with a dog. Come on, Nancy, Larry put you up to this didn't he?" Alice weighed in on the subject.

"Nancy, you got us good."

"Truthfully, I've never spoken to Larry about the subject. But I did see a man at the turnoff walking a dog and we even waved to each other. Maybe he is someone visiting in the area."

I decided to laugh it off. Joe was pretty quick to add.

"No one visiting that I know of, maybe you're confused about where you saw the man?"

"Maybe, I also saw him clear as a bell yesterday."

Alice was quiet and stared into her cup. She looked up at me.

"How long have you known Larry and Beth?"

"About twenty plus years, we've been neighbors in Phoenix."

"Beth and I were childhood friends. We have known each other forever. Both of us were born into old school Irish families. Irish families in Strawberry looked out for each other. My family had no money and Beth's father, in kindness, arranged for my family to rent very cheaply a small piece of his land on the outskirts of his parcel. My mother helped to look after Beth and her siblings after Beth's mother died. When Beth's father died our little piece of the parcel was willed to my mother. And we are on it today."

We all paused in the stillness; it felt heavy in the room.

"Yes," said Alice proudly, "the Irish looked out for each other. My family was so very grateful. There is nothing we wouldn't do for Larry and Beth."

My questions continued.

"Do you remember Beth's father's name?"

"I'm not sure, I have cobwebs in my brain sometimes, but I believe it was Patrick."

Bingo was all I could think. It made sense, the manuscript was telling the truth. It felt as if I had hit a jackpot or solved a mystery. Only I had to keep it to myself. I leaned toward Alice and cradled the warm cup in my hand and engaged her eyes.

"That is a good solid Irish name."

"More coffee Nancy? Are you warm enough?"

"Yes and yes. Let me get my own cup, I'd like a little milk in it."

"Why didn't you tell us that, we'd have given you some milk?"

"I like my first few cups black. It wakes me up."

I returned and settled back on their couch with my fourth cup of coffee. Joe started talking about living in a small town.

"A lot of strange things, people say, happen in small towns. Some claim they see ghosts or spirits."

I delighted in the turn of the conversation.

"But I don't pay any attention to ghost stuff, its hog wash. If you ask me I think the old Irish would say it was blarney."

Alice's reaction got my attention. She just smiled and drank her coffee. Again she turned her attention to me.

"Nancy, after you finish your coffee let's you and I go into my studio. If you are not in a hurry, I want to show you some of my paintings and then we can spirit talk. Joe doesn't like the subject of spirits, but I do. Then dear," she turned to Joe, "while Nancy and I talk you can finish your project in the shed."

"You women."

I could tell he just loved Alice to no end. It was obvious. People who have different philosophies appreciate one another for who they are. Joe and Alice were precious together.

"Joe is an electrical engineer."

And of course Joe added. "Alice is the artist."

"We exercise different sides of the brain."

This was going to be interesting. "I'm happy to stay and visit in the studio with you, Alice."

Joe buttoned up his coat and opened the back door to leave.

"If I see any tree fairies I'll call you both to come outside."

With that he slammed the door. Alice and I laughed. I stood up and took Alice's and my empty cups to the kitchen. When I returned Alice led me to her studio. There were lots of paintings.

"Most of them are of this house, our home in Strawberry, rather than of our other home in Tucson." She hesitated. "I don't believe in ghosts Nancy, but there is energy here on this land that I feel. The energy is comforting to me. Remember when you first walked into the kitchen and you said it felt like the house embraced you?"

I nodded.

"Well, I feel that peace and comfort here on this land in this house. You know the old Irish talked about the leprechauns. My mother would talk about the tree fairies in Ireland. My mother had the gift of gab."

I kept my focus on Alice's tree paintings. I told Alice about my beginning watercolor art class and the tree nymph that I painted. Alice looked amused.

"Really Alice, we splattered India ink on paper. Then we looked at the splatter and painted what we saw that came out of the splatter. Mine is a tree nymph."

Alice smiled from one side of her face to the other.

"That's great, dear."

I felt a kindred spirit in Alice. She could call me dear anytime. There was one thought Alice kept repeating during our conversation.

"There is so much we don't know, what we don't know does matter. Lead a good compassionate life and be kind to others, those are the things that matter."

We smiled at each other. I decided to stop with my questions about the old man walking his dog. I shifted the conversation.

"How did you and Joe meet? And specifically what is your secret for having a long and a wonderful marriage."

Alice began and told me she was born in Prescott, Arizona. Prescott was the capitol and the hot spot of Arizona. Alice's father was a teamster and her mother ran a boarding house there in Prescott. As best as Alice could remember "it was soooo long ago" her father was set up by enemies and got in trouble with the law. He was framed for something he didn't do. He packed up his family in the wee hours of the morning and headed for Payson, Arizona for a fresh beginning.

"You have to remember, Nancy, at that time Payson was a long way off. Today someone can drive it in a matter of a couple of hours. Back then it was treacherous and far away. Things change don't they?"

"Yes, some things change, like driving to Payson on an easy road, but framing someone for a crime he didn't commit still continues today, wouldn't you say?" It upsets me to hear injustices. But Alice just shifted her weight and nodded. I was sure Alice dealt with any emotions long ago. I wanted to dig a little deeper. "Of what crime was your father accused?"

"I may have heard it at one time, but I don't remember. If I had to guess I'd say a land dispute or a drunken brawl in a bar. The Irish liked to drink and they liked music. My father was no exception. In Ireland the bars are family places and everyone sings and dances. Have you been to Ireland, Nancy?"

"Yes and I loved it."

Alice spoke to me in her finest Irish brogue.

"Then ye know about the fairies especially in county Dingle?"

We both laughed and I vehemently shook my head yes.

"Then you know the roots of the mystical Ireland?"

I nodded. Alice explained how she said a prayer before she began any painting. She blessed the paint, the brushes, and the canvas.

"You know Nancy, privately, I discuss the mystical with individuals. Joe doesn't care to discuss or even listen to the mystical. I respect his wishes and stay clear of those conversations with him. You understand?"

"Of course."

"It is important for us to respect our differences. A lot of the people I knew as newlyweds through the years tried unsuccessfully to change their spouses. Each one thinks getting married will change the other person. If a person thinks her spouse is going to change she has a recipe for disaster. Would you want to be changed Nancy by someone who is telling you they love you?"

"Of course not."

"What is it that a person is saying if in one breath it's I love you and in the next breath it's I want to change you? I don't get it. I don't have to. It is none of my business."

"I never thought of it in that way. What you are saying makes sense."

Alice was lighthearted and a deep thinker.

"When Joe and I met at the Catholic Church in Prescott we were very young and both shy. Yet we knew to respect one another and our differences even back then. I didn't know anything about being assertive or any of that, I knew that I loved the essence of this man. Joe is hard working with a fabulous sense of humor that I am sure you saw today. He loves his family, maybe not above his God, but he loves his family. You know Nancy, we laugh all the time."

Then Alice wanted to know if I had ever married. Here we go, I thought, into judgment.

"No, close to it though several times. It seems I loved the ones who didn't love me or vice a versa. I just didn't hit the right page at the right time. My life is serial monogamy, but there is a level of intimacy that marriage teaches that I am missing. I don't believe all married people are intimate, not by a long shot. But many are and that is great. In other words intimacy doesn't always follow marriage."

Alice shook her head in agreement.

"Marriage is a long road, but worth the journey." She returned to her family history.

"My father came the back way from Prescott to Strawberry. When he arrived at the prearranged meeting site at the Catholic

Church in Strawberry, the priest suggested he could find work with a parishioner who had small children and had just lost his wife. It was a Godsend for my parents. The parishioner was Beth's father. The two men, Beth's father and my father became fast friends. Beth and I, of course, always played together."

Light bulbs went off in my head at Alice's words. I just smiled and drank it all in. After a minute of pause Alice continued.

"When I got older my mother took me to look at schools in Prescott. The priest arranged for me to stay in a parishioner's home and there I saw Joe for the first time. He did yard work for his uncle across the street. We actually met at church. Joe and I haven't been apart since." Alice wanted to make sure I knew marriage wasn't an easy road. "With a person like Joe it is worth every last bump."

"Alice I think you are a passionate person and create passion wherever you go."

"Nancy there is passion in painting and passion in loving. If you lose the passion in either then it is best to begin again somewhere else. Now mind you, not necessarily with a new man, but perhaps on a different path with the same man. It is like instead of painting in oil I can paint in watercolor, still painting, but a different path. You will see, Nancy."

"Maybe next lifetime, I am very content and my life is full right now. Intimacy with the right man would make it more interesting, but I am not complaining. I am happy."

I told Alice about the workshop I took on Real Love with Greg Baer.

"I love the concept that if one is so full of love there is nothing to interrupt or take away from that love."

The example Greg used is if you have a million dollars and someone steals two dollars off the kitchen table do you care? No, but if you only possess two dollars and someone steals it, you care very much. It is the same principal; if one is full of love then the little things are of no concern. Anything that is not love is a little thing. I may not be doing Greg's philosophy justice, but I put it out there. It is what I heard in the workshop anyway."

Alice looked interested and amused. Just then Joe came in the back door.

"Alice can you please get me a band aid? I finished in the shed, but I nicked my knuckle." Alice, like a nurse, put the band-aid over his knuckle. It was getting late for me.

'It's getting to be time for me to go and head back over to Larry and Beth's cabin." I was sure my disappointment showed. Alice and I smiled at each other.

I made my way through their house and found my coat. I made sure to pet the dog goodbye. We three humans exchanged hugs and said our good-byes. Joe gave a yell.

"Come back next year. Give Larry and Beth our love will you?"

"You bet."

I got in my car and traveled the now familiar road to Larry's cabin. My stomach and heart were both warm and full. My mind was clicking like a well-oiled clock. My thoughts returned to our breakfast conversation about the old man and his dog. I was a fan of Silvia Browne; the TV shows Medium, and Ghost Whisperer. Part of my mind was trying to convince me the man with his dog that I saw was a visitor in the area. Another part of my brain thought he could be a ghost with a ghost dog. I concluded it didn't really matter. It was what it was.

Chapter 35

Leaving the Cabin

Out of habit the folders came to my mind. The only one left uncompleted was the red one. Maybe I could try to dig behind the shed. No, I negated the idea. I reminded myself that Larry indicated it was optional. Maybe the red folder could become a good excuse to return to the cabin next summer. That would be cool. If I came back then I could visit with Joe and Alice. I could bring up my tree nymph painting to show Alice. I knew everything would work out if I trusted. I mused to myself. My mind jetted to the future and I thought about getting a dog and naming the dog Trust. I must be overly tired and overly stimulated at the same time. My best option was either to rest or to meditate. First I wanted to make a decision on staying another night in the cabin or not. My decision was quick and it was a no, it was time to go.

It was after one pm when I unlocked the cabin door and looked at the clock. First I wanted to collect the folders, check them one more time, and pack them making sure everything was there and accounted for. As that was completed I carefully put the box with the folders in my jeep. Next I began cleaning the cabin. If time permitted I could re-read the manuscript for a second time at a slower pace and savor the contents. As it turned out time didn't permit it. I opted to re-read the manuscript at the Strawberry Lodge after dinner. It was a good game plan that would get me out of the cabin and on the road by four pm. It took me longer than expected to clean the fireplace. I was amazed at the mess I had made in the past twenty-four-hour period. I finished the cleaning and was somewhat disappointed that I didn't have time to re-read the manuscript in the cabin. It had been precious reading it for the first time last night in this cabin. I doubted that I would ever forget it. I made one last round to check the locks on the windows and then I called Joe.

"Hi Joe, it's Nancy across the way, can you come over and disconnect the propane tank? Is now or later better for you? I am getting ready to go back to the lodge."

"I am on my way; hold tight till I get there."

Joe was at the door within ten minutes. Tucked under his arm was a small package he handed to me.

"Alice and I thoroughly enjoyed your company this morning. Alice wants you to have this."

The package was wrapped in old newspapers.

"Thank you both." I carefully opened the layers of newspaper. Inside was a painting Alice had painted of Larry and Beth's cabin.

"It is an old painting; one Alice did years ago. Alice must really like you because she generally keeps her old paintings. I know Alice definitely likes this one, it is one of her favorites."

"I am touched." This was all I could get out of my mouth. "Joe, could you please give me your mailing address in Tucson?"

Joe smiled as he handed me a piece of paper with the information already on it.

"Thank you Joe and thank Alice, please."

We hugged. Joe went out the door and around the back of the cabin to disconnect the propane tank. Two minutes later he was in his car, waved to me, and drove off.

I obsessed about this cabin being clean, locked, and everything turned off. Finally, after triple checks, I pulled out of the driveway. I glanced back at the cabin in my rear view mirror. I wanted to return next year. The snow from last night was mostly melted and it was sunny and clear. The ride back to the motel was uneventful. I kept looking for the old man and the dog but saw nothing. I didn't even see a coyote.

It was just beginning to get dark as I pulled into a parking space at the lodge. My room looked the same; everything was just as I had left it. It looked the same, but I was different. I placed the box with the folders on the nightstand. I pulled out the yellow folder and placed the manuscript on the bed. For the next fifteen minutes I meditated.

My stomach growled with hunger pangs. I decided on an early dinner. Anything except granola bars would be good. I locked the door and took the steps that led to the dining room. There was a big chandelier in the dining room and some elk heads on the wall. Pictures of the people who started the Strawberry Lodge were framed on the walls. It was authentic Strawberry. I sat myself at a booth and drooled at the menu. The waitress approached.

"Where have you been?" It was a friendly banter and not nosy. I felt comfortable being open. I was a regular.

"I've been helping my Phoenix neighbors with their cabin down the road here." I pointed to the menu and ordered baked fish with macaroni and cheese. It was a carb high but so what. I knew I would finish my meal tonight with a cup of coffee and some dessert. It became peach pie and coffee. When the waitress placed my bill in front of me I felt pretty brave.

"Do you know who that old man is who walks his dog? I generally see him around the Old School House turnoff."

"Don't tell me you saw him?" She laughed out loud.

"What's so funny about that?" I must have looked shocked.

"You know it could be anybody with a dog but there is, and has been, a rumor for many years or maybe even decades now that there is a ghost walking a ghost dog. He is supposed to be wearing a cowboy hat. Rumor has it that the man lived in this area. No one knows and I don't care."

I just smiled.

"Who knows?" The waitress turned to go back into the kitchen. I couldn't wait to get back to my room and re-read the manuscript.

Chapter 36

Last Night at the Motel

After dinner I stopped by the front desk to let them know this was my last night. I gave her my charge card for the bill. The same woman who checked me in when I arrived checked me out.

"How was your room? Everything okay?"

"It was great." I felt brave. "Do you have any ghost stories in Strawberry?"

"No, I don't pay attention to that stuff. You sleep well tonight and come back and see us. I heard you were helping our Larry and Beth. They are great people. I was in Beth's Sunday school class up here, years ago. She didn't remember me last time they were in for dinner last summer. She remembered my sister though and called her by name." Another customer came in and her attention shifted. "You take care, Nancy."

I knew I would return in summer, the place was homey, they were friends of my neighbors and they knew my name, Nancy.

"Thanks for everything, I'll be back."

I returned to my room and changed into my pajamas. My flannel pajamas felt extra soft and warm since I was without last night. I climbed into the large bed, turned on the reading lamp, and picked up the folders. I started with the newspaper clip-pings. I was afraid to touch them for fear of tearing them; they were so old and crumpled. To my surprise there were pictures of pamphlets on Solidarity, on Sabotage, the IWW, and what they stood for. The print was old, water damaged, and just too fragile. I placed the clippings gently back in the folder for Larry to review in Phoenix. I decided it was wiser and more interesting to re-read the manuscript for a second time. I snuggled in the bed. The next thing I knew I heard doors slam. My first reaction was I'm in a cabin alone. Then it hit me; no, I had fallen asleep reading in my bed and I was at the Strawberry Lodge. Knowing I was safe in the lodge I placed the manuscript on the nightstand, rolled over and went back to sleep. I dreamt, but didn't remember what.

The clock on the nightstand said nine and the sun was out. I spent a few more minutes under the blanket, and reviewed the past couple of days. I savored the memory. I got out of bed, show-ered, and welcomed the day. My meditation was ten minutes. I was anxious to get on the road. I could meditate more over my morning coffee.

Chapter 37

On the Road Home

I was in my Jeep, a Strawberry Lodge coffee cup in hand, by ten AM. The song "On the Road Again" was playing in my head. No matter where I traveled or what I did, it always felt good to head home. I imagined it was the same for everyone. My camera was in the front seat and I drove through Payson, which is known for its beautiful views of the rim and trees. It was an optimum time to go on a picture-taking escapade. The weather was perfect and clear. A cool crispness was in the air. Coolness was always welcome to this Phoenician. Larry crossed my mind and I decided to give him a call. I didn't want to discuss the manuscript over the phone. I didn't know how I would approach the subject of my reading the manuscript, but I knew I would tell him. I trusted. Guilt crept in. When I picked up my phone the message beeper was activated. I had forgotten to check for messages. There was one message, which ended up being a sales call. I called my neighbor, JJ, who wasn't home. I left a message letting him know I was on my way home to Phoenix.

Up ahead was the Denny's restaurant that I had stopped at on my way up to Strawberry. I wasn't hungry, but I wanted the experience of being called Annie again. I pulled in the same parking spot and entered the front door. It was a different hostess, but the same waiter. The hostess welcomed me, but didn't ask my name. I was disappointed. I wanted to respond my name is Annie.

I ended up with the same waiter who remembered me, but not my name. I laughed to myself. I could be Annie right now, but no one knew it. I ordered iced tea and vegetable soup. Aside from not being able to say Annie, being in the restaurant didn't feel any different. I knew that either as Annie or Nancy my thoughts were loving and supportive. Those loving and supportive thoughts set the tone for my trip. It had nothing to do with my identity or a name I called myself. It had to do with my intention. What I focused my attention on was where I was. At the time it must have been easier for me to call it Annie rather than an intention. It worked.

Metaphysics was interesting to me. A person got to be creative and responsible. Like being a snowflake with the gift of awareness and intention that floated in the middle of New York City. Some snowflakes in New York City crashed against the sides of tall buildings and some rested on trees, but the snowflake aware of its source was always at peace. Peace was a choice. The geographic location was not responsible for the journey. An aware snowflake decided on being scared or sacred. I was grateful for my journey and my freedom. In more ways than one it was time for me to move on. I paid my bill and left a nice tip. As I left Denny's the hostess from my previous visit arrived for her shift. She waved and called out to me.

"Hi Annie, good to see you."

Startled and speechless would be an understatement. The hostess was like my long lost old friend.

"You know Annie, you look so much like my niece in Indiana named Annie that I could just swear you are her twin." The hostess turned for the bathroom and was out of my sight. I laughed and continued out the door to my car.

Payson was a relaxing stop for me. I pulled off the road at Woods Canyon Lake and meditated under a tree in the dense woodlands. The smell of pine trees was refreshing and the breeze rustled the leaves. It felt mystical to me. Pictures couldn't do justice to the Rim. I decided to just lean against a tree and soak it all in. I remembered an old Native American belief I had heard years ago; talk your problems into a rock, place the rock under a tree, and the energy of the tree transfers your negative energy into positive. For many years I had heard that if one was in the woods and needed energy, one could lean against an old tree and receive energy from the tree. Trees were a magnificent power. Once, when I was in California at the Asilomar state park I meditated under a tree. I felt as if I went inside the tree; I flowed and sensed the flow of nutrients move up and down the trunk of the tree. It was enlightening. Nature is a beautiful teacher. I began to feel anxious and it was time to leave the forest and return to Phoenix.

Chapter 38

Phoenix

It was dark when I arrived in Phoenix. As I unlocked the front door my cat, Tweetie, meowed in protest at my absence. First things first, I fed Tweetie. There wasn't much for me to unpack. The precious manuscript was neatly re-tied with the old string and rested in the yellow folder. I looked out my side window to see if a light was on at Larry and Beth's house. Maybe it would be better to talk to Larry in the daytime. I saw a light on in their kitchen and called. No one answered. I left a message that I was back from Strawberry and to give me a call when he had time. As an after thought I decided tomorrow would be a good day to visit Beth and hopefully she was out of the Intensive Care Unit.

About a half an hour later my phone rang and it was Larry.

"I'm glad your back and had a safe trip." His voice sounded weak or tired. "Are you free tomorrow morning Nancy, maybe we can have coffee?"

"Sure, that sounds great. How is Beth doing?"

"She is much better and may be discharged from the hospital. The doctors are deciding if a care facility would be better than home for the next few days. It may be awhile before she is able to come home."

I knew Larry would explain more in the morning, but he sounded exhausted.

"Would you like me to bring some bagels to go with the coffee?"

"If you like, Nancy."

The next morning I awoke with a strong desire to hike my healing mountain, but it would have to wait as too much was going on. Morning was my favorite time to hike, maybe tomorrow. Larry called around nine and suggested I come over.

"Great." And I was on my way. My hands were full with the box of folders, the weed eater, frozen bagels, and the shovel. Larry heard me before he saw me.

"Oh Nancy, I needed a good laugh." He opened the door and took the shovel out of my hands.

"The shovel was just in case you wanted to dig up the box by the shed. In the old days people didn't have banks or didn't trust in banks. They would hide their cash under a mattress or bury it." He explained further that the box contained several hundred dollars in cash for emergencies.

"Except now a couple hundred dollars wouldn't help you too much."

He looked inside the box with the folders. He picked up the first folder, the orange one with the house key and the map. He carefully looked through the remaining folders; the green folder containing the old faded envelope with the title, the blue folder with the personal papers; the white folder with the key to the shed; the red folder with the information on digging up the "basement level box" and the yellow folder with the manuscript. I'm not sure if it was my imagination, but I swore Larry looked at me with eyes that said you read the manuscript didn't you?

"Yes I read it." I blurted. I never could keep a secret for long. Relief must have been on my face. Larry laughed.

"I would have guessed you'd read it."

"So, is the manuscript true? Why all the secrecy?"

"Is what true?"

"Was Patrick your father in law?"

"Maybe." Larry was coy. He was a very intelligent man who wasn't giving an inch. I went on.

"Was there really a dog named Trust? Did you really see a dog and man walking on the property? Do you think they are ghosts? Do you believe in ghosts?"

Larry was saved by the bell. His phone rang. It was Beth wanting to know where he was and why he was late. I overheard Larry's side of the conversation.

"Nancy is here and we are going over a few things. I'll be there shortly, dear. Beth, are you ready for some visitors? Nancy wants to visit you."

I didn't hear Beth's response, but I could hear Larry.

"I'll tell Nancy not to visit you today, maybe later in the week you would like some company."

They spoke a few more minutes and then he ended their conversation.

"I love you, sweetie."

Larry returned to the room and looked deep in thought. I prayed that he wasn't mad or upset at me for reading the manuscript.

"Larry, I apologize for reading something that clearly wasn't for my eyes."

"No, no, no, it's not that. For years I wanted someone to read it and now someone has. I want to know what you think. It is true. Beth's father is Patrick and Patrick swore me to secrecy. To this day Beth has very little knowledge that the manuscript exists and what it documents. He didn't want to endanger anyone. Her whole life her father, Patrick, told her he was a farmer. He was a grand man. I never met Beth's mother, she passed away when Beth was small. Of course when I first met Patrick I was scared to death of him yet I always knew he was in my corner. He was very supportive. When he was getting very sick and dying he swore me to secrecy and told me the story. The interesting thing is he always had dogs and every one of them was named Trust. He would tell people he named all his dogs the same so he wouldn't forget their name. He was a grand man. Did you open the envelope in the green folder, the title?"

"No, I was respectful there."

He looked me straight in the eyes.

"I trusted you to do the right thing and you did. You didn't give it to anyone but me. I think subconsciously I wanted you to read it. Here look at this envelope, the one with the title; I haven't looked at any of this in years. I wasn't sure it would all be there. I don't know whom I thought would take it or if I thought it would disintegrate. Patrick was a prince of a man and I respected him as he respected me."

I felt guilty that I may have violated Patrick and Larry's privacy. Larry's word eased my guilty conscience.

"I am glad you read it, it is important to me that it was read. The kids are all out of town, and you are a dear to us."

He had the old envelope in his hand and opened it. His wrinkled strong hands on the old fragile envelope fascinated me. It was a picture of a thousand words. My camera was at my house next door, but then again a camera would have spoiled the moment. He pulled out this old yellow paper from the envelope and handed it to me. I could barely make out the print, but I saw the name Al and the name Patrick. I knew it had to be the official deed or transfer of title from so long ago. It had to be the actual one that Al had arranged for Patrick to sign in Prescott, just as it was told in the manuscript.

"Patrick was a very easy going, hard working man who loved his family and his dogs. The only time I ever saw fear in Patrick's eyes was when he reminisced about the unions and his buddy Al. Patrick made me swear never to discuss Jerome with Beth. Now you are in the loop Nancy and it is old information. You know Nancy, I could tell Patrick didn't want to discuss Jerome with me, but he said at the time he had to tell someone. Patrick told me he thought Al was probably dead by then and no one would ever hear from him. Patrick wanted me at all costs to honor Al's request for secrecy, and I have honored his request." Larry paused a minute.

It only took me two seconds to promise Patrick I would keep the secret.

Larry turned to me. "The time has come for me to tell someone and I must ask you, as Patrick asked me, to keep the secret."

I was speechless and deeply honored. I looked at him.

"You have my word."

Larry reached out his hand and we shook. I knew it was more than a handshake, I knew it was the proverbial gentleman's handshake. Larry broke the silence.

"Now there is one more business matter. You know our children and grandchildren live so far away, would you someday be interested in purchasing our cabin in Strawberry? Beth and I will make sure it is a good price and one that you can afford. We would like it to be with someone who will use it. Our kids live too far away and would probably just turn around and sell it. What do you think, Nancy?"

I was flattered and my heart skipped a beat. Larry was offering me a treasure from their life. It would be fun, but I would have to think it through. That was what tomorrows were for, to think things through. My arms reached to Larry and we hugged.

"What a wonderful thought Larry; I know how much that cabin means in your lives. Let me think about it. And besides you might not be selling it for a long time."

"Good. Let me discuss it with Beth and the kids; you know both Beth and I are approaching ninety and our cabin days may be ending. With Beth's medical condition I am not sure we will go this summer and if we do, how long we will be there. I will keep you posted. Remember Nancy I have your word that no matter what happens you will keep the secret."

"You have my word. Even though I didn't fully understand it, it was a beautiful story. I won't share the information with another human being."

Larry opened the door to let me out and say good night.

"I believe the spirit of Patrick and his dog are talking to me now, reminding me to trust."

"Me too. Goodbye, Larry."

We hugged and Larry hurried off to be with Beth.

Chapter 39

Hiking

It was still early in the day and I headed off for my healing mountain. The heck with doing the wash and going to the grocery store, I was retired and could take my good ole time, echoed in my mind. There were plenty of water bottles still in my cooler from my trip. And, of course, my hiking boots were always in the jeep. I was off. It was an overcast day with some wind. Consistent sunny days for weeks on end wore me down. The past summer had been hot. I was grateful for a change to coolness; windy and overcast was great.

I didn't know why it felt so good to hike and why it always felt better to hike this mountain than any other mountain in Phoenix. I concluded it was because consciously and subconsciously I had learned a lot about myself on this mountain. It was why I even named it the healing mountain. There was something about this mountain, at least for me. I wanted to know what the mountains knew. The old phrase, if these walls could talk, kept popping up in my mind. If only these rocks on the mountain could talk. It wasn't just the existence of energy on this mountain that gave me something. It was some kind of energy exchange or as I would say to Ted, my hiking buddy, this mountain accepted me, all of me, in my most rugged form. It couldn't very well kick me off the mountain. It was unconditional acceptance. The exchange was acceptance. Now that was a teaching. I imagined Ted's laughter.

In the past he and I had shared some very deep secrets on this mountain.

Maybe it was my intention. I intended to love and honor this mountain. I looked around and there was Ted. I had passed many people on the trail today. It was a beautiful day. Most of the people I didn't know. The regulars hiked early in the day, and it was almost noon. Ted saw me.

"You are here late. How was your trip?"

"Better than expected."

"I want to hear about it, but I have a Doctor's appointment and I am late. I'll see you up here next week and we can catch up."

We hugged. He continued down while I hiked on up the mountain.

After hiking I stopped by the store for some fresh salad makings and headed home. It was gradually getting darker and colder in Phoenix. It was actually below fifty-five degrees. This was fireplace weather in Phoenix.

The Christmas season was approaching. It was an exceptional time for gratitude.

The following week I visited Beth in the convalescent home. She was preparing to come home in a couple of days and was in the best of spirits. I was her only company for the afternoon. Larry was out running errands. She greeted me with a big hug.

"Larry told me story of how my father got the cabin in Strawberry. I always wondered how we ended up in Strawberry; it is such a small town. My mother would say it is a good place for immigrants. It was a rugged lifestyle as were most lifestyles in that time period."

"Beth what is your favorite story about your father, Patrick?"

She got a tear in her eye.

"One winter about two feet of snow had fallen and it was too deep for our little feet even with boots on. With that much snow Father would lead us children to school. He would put his big boot in the snow and make a big indentation. We would follow behind and place our little boots inside the indentations his big boots left. He made it easier for us to get to school. We didn't have to push so hard on the snow with our little boots. Our little legs weren't that strong. He did that for us. He was a kind man."

"Very kind." I knew Beth had many stories. One thing she remembered was that her mother had lost her first-born son at birth.

"They were going to name their first born Albert. You know Nancy in the old days people lost their children in birth and no one talked about it. Then when my mother died my father lost his best friend. He never looked at another woman. He would read to us each evening and tuck us in with a kiss. He would always tell us to remember your mother is watching over you. She is in the clouds and in the sunshine. He would always end with a kiss and the question, what is the one word I want you to remember your whole life?" Beth giggled.

"And we would each yell out 'trust' as loud as we could. You know I had forgotton about that word "trust" and all his dogs. I don't know how many dogs, I think five or six and they were all named Trust. My father was a wonderful man."

"I never met him, but would agree. I wish I would have met him."

Beth was grateful for my visit.

"Thank you Nancy for letting me remember such fond memories of my father, treasures really. When I get back home I promise to find the old pictures so you can see. There aren't many of them left and what is left are on tin plates." Beth was sure there was one of Patrick, her father.

"Give me a few months to get back on my feet. Maybe I will even take another trip with you to Strawberry."

"Now that would be exciting, Beth."

I asked Beth a few more questions about the copper mines in Jerome. Beth couldn't remember much about any mining stories. All she remembered was one time some one was praising the men who owned the coal mines in front of her father. It was one of the few times Beth ever saw her father get red in the face with anger.

"I don't honestly remember what was said just that my father got very angry, which startled me at the time." Beth remembered hearing stories of her father connecting with Catholic Churches for referrals. And she remembered hearing something about Appalachia.

"Nancy when you were reading did you read the name Elizabeth anywhere?" Beth's given name at birth was Elizabeth, which was shortened to Beth. Beth didn't know for whom she was named. As a child, she remembered she had asked, but was told it was just a pretty name her mother had liked. Beth always wondered because the other children were named for specific people.

Beth asked about my visit with Joe and Alice. She reminded me that she and Alice had been friends since childhood. She told me the history of Alice's artwork and that it was very much sought after. I told her about the painting Alice had given me as a gift, a painting of Larry and Beth's cabin. Beth was delighted and surprised. She suggested that I get to know Alice better. Alice was a very spiritual person. She loved the land and art.

Section III

The Sequel;
Claiming the Sacred in
Every Minute

Christmas

Christmas was wonderful and enchanting shared with extended family and friends. The smell of pine candles permeated my home. It was a wonderful time in Phoenix with picture perfect weather. The day after Christmas was full of my favorite leftovers and laughter. I visited Beth several times in the hospital and once after she had returned home. Larry called me and invited me over for a cup of tea. When I got there he looked a bit sad.

"My girls want the cabin. Beth and I were surprised by their reaction when we told them we wanted to sell it. Who would have guessed they were interested in it. I'm sorry Nancy if we disappointed you."

"Not to worry Larry, I am glad they want it, the cabin belongs in your family."

He and Beth had to be happy the kids and their families felt a connection to the cabin. The family decided to come together in the New Year to celebrate Beth being home. There would be a family dinner and Larry wanted me there. At the dinner Larry planned on transferring the title and more importantly talking about the history of the cabin, and especially about Patrick.

"I really want you at the dinner Nancy so you can share your experience."

"I am delighted. Larry, I feel relief, I didn't know how I would take care of a cabin, I have enough challenge with my house. It all works out when we trust. Doesn't it?"

We grinned at each other.

"Oh by the way Larry, don't forget to have the electricity turned off in the cabin. Joe and Alice wanted me to remind you."

This was the first time Larry and I had a chance to talk about my breakfast with Joe and Alice.

"In summary meeting Joe and Alice was all good and all fun."

Family Dinner

The family dinner was at Beefeaters on West Camelback Road in Phoenix. It was an old fashioned elegant restaurant. Everyone was jovial and full of expectation. Beth was using a walker and ready for a fun evening. It was lovely seeing the daughters with their spouses and families. Fun was the theme of the evening. Larry had asked me to type and make copies of the manuscript to distribute at the family dinner.

After dessert everyone got quiet and Larry pulled out the deed for transfer. He had all the work prepared for the daughters' signatures. They both signed. He showed everyone the original deed complete with Al's address in Jerome. Then he pulled out the yellow folder now stuffed with the original manuscripts plus copies of the manuscript. He began his speech and held up the original.

"I wrote this over fifty years ago. During the past couple of weeks Beth and I have read and re-read this story. It is about an old man and his dog. It is the history of how Beth's father, your grandfather, Patrick came to Strawberry." The room was silent. "I will give you each a copy, take your time and read it." Larry gave a brief synopsis of Patrick's history. "Nancy was just there at the cabin. She picked up the documents for me and typed the manuscript. I thank her for that."

There was a mysterious air in the room.

"Don't read it now but at your leisure, that is, if you even want to read it. Tonight is for fun. Set the story aside." Larry suggested the family invite me to the cabin. "Nancy has met and now knows our old friends, Joe and Alice."

The family invited me to the cabin anytime I wanted to go. They wanted me to at least pick a week that could be my week each year. I could have the cabin to myself. It didn't take me long to reply in the affirmative.

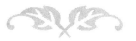

Jerome

The week after New Year's Day I drove the hour and half ride up to Jerome for lunch. On the way up I recalled all the times in the past twenty five years that I had taken guests from out of state to Jerome. They all loved the little ghost town. For drama I included a story about the sheriff of Jerome arrested for smoking pot back in the sixties or seventies. I wasn't sure if I had read or heard it. The story confirmed to my visitors that the Wild West was still wild.

I was always drawn to the town of Jerome, but not necessarily to the museum. I preferred to be outdoors. When I took guests to Jerome invariably one of them would read out loud the description of Jerome from the AAA book:

In 1582 Spanish missionaries exploring the Verde Valley recorded that natives were using the copper mines near what is now Jerome. The missionaries' description of the mines was identical to the workings found in 1883 by the United Verde Co. Eugene Jerome of New York agreed to finance the mining project on condition the camp be named for him. In 1886 a smelter arrived by rail from Ash Fork and operations began in earnest.

Once a city with a population of 15,000, Jerome became a virtual ghost town when the United Verde Branch copper mines of the Phelps

Dodge Corp closed in 1953.since then shops, galleries, studios and museums have been established in the restored town. Some of the restored homes are open during the Home Tour in May.

Jerome State Historic Park is off SR 89A. The Park Museum in the 1916 adobe brick Douglas mansion traces the history of local mining and the family of James S. Douglas, developer of the rich United Verde Extension Mine in the early 1900s. A movie highlighting the history of Jerome is shown continuously. Picnicking is permitted.

By design I took this trip by myself. At Larry's house, he had shown me the original deed signed by Al and Patrick. I couldn't read the last names, but I did read the return address, which was in Jerome. When I reached Jerome I headed straight for the main street through town rather than taking the turnoff to the mine museum. I wandered around the town and peeked in at some of the galleries. I had a general idea of the return address, which I thought might have been Al's house. To my amazement a structure or what was left of a structure set at the address. It was obvious no one at present lived there. The appearance didn't matter; it was the history that made the address important to me. Too bad I didn't have any address for the rooming house Patrick had stayed in back in the early 1900s. The House of Joy was easy to locate with its ornate banister. The House of Joy remained in shape through the years because it was business store and a restaurant. Looking at the ornate railings on the outside of the building I imagined the prostitutes and men literally hanging over the sides.

I walked down the street a little more. The view from the edge of town was breathtaking. It looked over the mine and in the distance the red rocks of Sedona were visible. It had to be rough living up here for those miners especially without any family support. Up in these mountains it appeared to be desolate. As I visited galleries and shops I would ask about ghost stories. As expected there were several ghost stories in the area. Two were of resident ghosts who had died in the old hospital now a hotel. The Arizona Republic newspaper was doing a story I was told. I continued to wander the area. It crossed my mind that the reporter for the ghost story could be the same reporter writing on my healing mountain. That would be a hoot. I stopped at the Asylum restaurant at the hotel. The lunch menu was gourmet. A wonderful strawberry pecan salad caught my eye. My little table was by a window that overlooked the valley. The view was worth a million dollars. After lunch I drove down to the museum. The views along the way were spectacular. I doubted if the early miners ever had the opportunity to enjoy views. With their long workdays I doubted they even saw the light of day above ground.

I drove around a circular driveway to the museum and parked. The museum was an old mansion just as the AAA book had indicated. I climbed the stairs and entered a back display room. I was startled. It had been years since I was at this museum. Generally when I came to Jerome it was for lunch, shopping, and hiking. Ahead of me in a glass case were multiple papers with information on the Jerome deportation. I recognized the pamphlets and wording on solidarity, sabotage and the IWW that I collected from Larry's cabin. Everything referenced in the manuscript was before my eyes in the glass case. It was all true. There was even a picture of some men in a cattle car. I would have to tell Beth and Larry. Wow, I thought, that could be a picture of Al and I just didn't know it. I had no idea what Al or Patrick looked like.

As long as I was in Jerome I ventured into questioning residents. A woman gardening told me about a research project on the Jerome deportation completed several years ago by a college student from back east. The student documented everything she had discovered and it became her thesis. No one remembered the student's name or the location of the research papers. It was thought that the display at the museum was a result of her research. The woman gardening said the researcher was affiliated with a university back east probably in Arkansas. A future project for me would be to email several universities and hope that someone could locate the thesis.

Beth would be a good one to identify old pictures of her father. I knew that it was highly unlikely that Patrick would be in any pictures because he was in town for such a short time, but it was worth a try I rationalized. I talked to a couple of park rangers in the vicinity. They gave me all sorts of information that included the name of someone in the Phoenix area knowledgeable about the Jerome deportation. The woman's name was Greta and she lived in Phoenix. The ranger thought Greta was around eight-five and sharp as a tack. She lived with her son who was a friend of the ranger. I thanked the rangers and left Jerome.

When I returned home I contacted Greta. She had a copy of the doctoral thesis on the Jerome Deportation completed by the student. The student's grandfather had lived in nearby Sedona. I visited Greta at home and was amazed at her knowledge of history for the Verde Valley area that included Jerome. She talked about the Jerome family spending their summers in England and how Jenny Jerome was connected to the Churchill family.

Eventually I turned the conversation to ghosts. Greta was interested.

"I've heard a lot of ghost stories particularly in the Jerome mine but I never saw a ghost myself." I felt disappointed, but Greta went on.

"I don't believe in ghosts, but if I did, my favorite tale is about an old man and sometimes two men. They are seen walking around the streets of Jerome, even today, leading up to the old mine. The old miners would whisper to me." Greta lowered her voice "the ghosts are those of a miner who was loyal to his convictions and wouldn't betray the workers. Some say the man was the manager for the mines. Supposedly he either died or was murdered in the mines for sticking up for his men. Sometimes he is seen walking with another man and a big black dog. No one knows a name but if you see them you can hear him call out one word, 'Trust.' Supposedly they call out trust like they are calling to someone. Some of the old timers say Trust was a dog, but who knows."

Greta got a huge smile on her face.

"Nancy did you know that God spelled backwards is dog? Are you okay Nancy? You look like you've seen a ghost."

"I'm fine just a little tired, I'll drink a little water." I pulled a small bottle of water out of my purse. "Actually Greta you aren't the first person to tell me about that ghost story. Did you say some people still see it?"

Greta nodded.

"Do you have any names of people who still see the ghost? I would love to speak with them."

Greta explained that most of the old timers were dead but there are still a couple of people in Jerome who could confirm the ghost story. They were good friendly people who might be willing to talk to me.

"It is a good thing that the doctoral student did her research on the Jerome Deportation and not on ghost stories. People would have been upset or fearful to talk about ghosts." Greta excused her self and went into the other room and brought back her address book. She wrote down some names and numbers for me and handed me the piece of paper with the phone numbers.

"These are three names and phone numbers with addresses."

"Thank you Greta, I am excited. I will be planning another trip to Jerome. Perhaps this time I'll spend a couple of nights there."

Greta suggested that I call her after my visits with the three people.

"In the interim Nancy I'll look for pictures. This is fun. I love to talk about Jerome."

We hugged and said our goodbyes.

Show Low

For several months the idea of owning land in Show Low percolated in my psyche. If not in Show Low then some other land in northern Arizona. I kept dreaming of Show Low. Sometime in February was the scheduled opening of ranch land near Show Low. In full gear I prepared for my next adventure and Show Low was the destination. My intention was becoming a mantra "I am revealing the sacred in the moment like a falling snowflake, nothing is permanent." It was as if I had retired into the sacredness that had always been there only I didn't know it.

On one of my last trips to Thunderbird Mountain Ted had caught up with me and we had climbed together. We talked about the newspaper article on the mountain. He had seen it also.

"It isn't a big deal." He really wanted to know something else. "Did you get to Show Low yet?"

"No, too much else going on, but in the near future I hope to change that."

"Now is a good time to visit Show Low. My granddaughter says there are lots of new real estate lots being developed and the prices are good. Some are thirty-six acre ranches. It sounded like a good idea to me. For the second time Ted gave me his granddaughter's name and phone number.

"Now call her when you get to Show Low."

"Thanks Ted." Inside I thought it was unlikely that I would call her. I didn't even know Ted's last name or phone number. We were mountain friends.

Later that day when I opened my mail there was a brochure for land in Show Low. I must have ordered it. Pictures on the front of the brochure featured some ancient pictographs carved into the stones right there on the land. The ancient stone etchings looked similar to the ones I had seen at Boynton Canyon in Sedona. I'd never looked for any ancient carvings on the healing mountain in Phoenix, but maybe they were there. I needed to explore. They may be off the beaten track and I would have to be careful not to destroy the balance of nature.

George called and wanted to hike. We planned a trip to Show Low so I could look at the ranches. A ranch was something I'd thought about often. George supported the idea. He was, however, more interested in motor homes. Neither George nor I were knowledgeable in car mechanics, but we both were knowledgeable in freedom and responsibility. We found good mechanics for our cars. We could learn the ropes of a motor home. There was always the option of renting one. Many singles travel in groups. George informed me that there were motor home parks that catered to the gay population. He also shared that there was a group of single women who traveled together and wagoned around a central fire at night. It could be a Thelma and Louise moment for me. I might even look for shards of old pottery.

Journal Review

As a habit each December I review my journal. It was a good way to review and bring closure to my year. My philosophy was unfinished business weighed a person down. In retrospect some of my business was juvenile and dramatic to my eyes that were now a year older and wiser.

In the moment of recording feelings, they are real. Once expressed, they transition. My expressions of anger didn't have to be expressed to another person. I just had to un-repress any pent up emotion. Without some form of expression my feelings stayed repressed like an abscess and blocked happiness. When repression overloaded my system a volcano exploded. Journaling was a safe place to express. I knew that most of the time my journaling had nothing to do with the other person or people. It was all about my learning and healing. I repeated and wrote on a small index card "I am revealing the sacred in the moment like a falling snowflake, nothing is permanent." If I learned anything this year it was to trust.

There were several phrases of comfort that surfaced in my mind. I'd been blessed with many teachers along my way; some I had liked and some that I didn't. Still they were all teachers. Savoring the moment was a phrase I carried in times of joy. With all the business and fighting in the world, savoring the moment created enjoyment. To take a moment and breathe in that wonderful energy of air, to sense its freshness, to sense its nourishing presence in my lungs, was a gift to my body. In all my busyness I missed some beauty on a daily basis. In my freedom of retirement now was my time to focus and savor. Nothing was more important and more creative than appreciation in the moment. Choosing sacred or scared was a choice moment by moment. A favorite meditation tape began with a phrase that went something like "Where your attention is, there you are." I know the focus of my attention created more of the same. I could choose busyness or beauty. Thoughts create things. Thought precedes form. Their origin wasn't as important as was the implementation.

Many people would tell me to smell the roses when I was stressed out. I debunked a popular myth that retired people have nothing to be stressed about. Sometime I had stress about finances. I don't know that I will ever know when I have enough. In the scheme of things the most important thing to me was my spiritual growth. In the realm of eternity that was all that mattered. Outside of the planet earth, money was nothing. Spiritual currency was something else. Money in itself was good like chocolate, tea, and food. It was an effect, but it could be used for good or bad. It was a responsibility as was freedom. With freedom came responsibility. I trusted the integrity of my soul to get the healing I came to earth for. My words and experiences fell as a snowflake and stuck with me, "nothing is permanent everything is changing. I am revealing the sacred in this moment like a falling snowflake, nothing is permanent."

The Healing Mountain

Climbing a mountain, any mountain is the story. I compared climbing the mountain with living life. The top of the mountain is like the end of life; the real story is in the living or the journey up the mountain. However, when I reached the top I stopped to enjoy the view. I find it interesting that I rarely stopped on my way up to enjoy the view. Just as my life, in my earlier years, I was too busy to enjoy the view, now I realized the view was on the hike all the way up, at the top, and all the way down the mountain. I can say my healing mountain teaches me to savor the moment, to remember to savor the view along my way and not just the view at the top. There was no hurry. I was free.

Usury Mountain

Frieda and Ben always went to Quartzite for the annual motor home get together. It was well advertised and thousands of people attended. Some came for the gem shows and others for the social aspect. Many times they had invited me, but I had declined. This time they insisted. They figured out a way for all of us to be comfortable. They stayed in their motor home and I in their travel trailer. It was extraordinarily kind.

I was ready for an adventure and we worked out the driving details. It was my first time sleeping in a camping trailer. They slept in their motor home. We hiked two days and hung out in the evenings around a campfire with other travelers. It was fun to meet the other motor home folks and we had a grand ole time. There is a camaraderie that exists among the motor home folks.

On our last hike we descended Usury Mountain. We passed a senior gentleman with his unleashed dog coming up the trail. The man greeted us as he passed.

"Hello."

Unbeknownst to the old man his dog had stopped to sniff me. I bent down and petted the dog. The dog was a friendly black lab with big beautiful eyes. The old man was about twenty yards ahead on the trail when he turned around and realized his dog was behind with me. He called down to his dog.

"Hurry up girl, come on girl, come on, Trust." Trust responded and ran up the trail to join him.

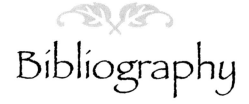

Bibliography

The Science of Mind Textbook / Ernest Holmes/ Jeremy P. Tarcher/Putnam a member of Penguin Putnam Inc./ 1938

Real Love / Greg Baer, M.D. /Gotham Books published by Penguin Group /2003

Man and his Symbols / Carl J. Jung / Aldus Books limited, London / 1964

Dream Power / Dr. Ann Faraday / Afar Publishing / 1972

Four Agreements / Don Miquel Ruiz / Amber Allen Publishing / 1997

Illuminata / Marianne Williamson /Random House / 1994

Who Dies / Stephen Levine / Anchor Books/ 1989

What The Bleep Do We Know / William Arntz, Betsy Chasse and Mark Vincent e/ Health Communications Inc / 2005

Radical Forgiveness / Colin C. Topping / Global 13 Publications, Inc / 1997

Juan Quezada / Shelly Dale / Norman Books / 2003

Payson Rim Country Relocation Guide / 2007/2008

Jerome Mining Museum / Arizona Labor Records

Arizona Republic Newspapers

The Power of Intention / Dr. Wayne W. Dyer / Hay House Inc. / 2004

The Road Less Traveled / M. Scott Peck / Touchstone SimonSchuster / 1978

About the Author

Nancy Lee Burns lives in Phoenix, Arizona and has called the desert home for thirty years. She is a self-described adventurer who recently retired from the field of social services. Her joys are writing, hiking, meditating, and painting icons. Her family and friends include numerous pets who reportedly call her "Auntie Nancy."

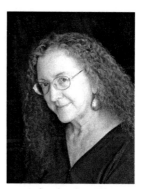

Author photo by Amy Kennedy

Her credentials include a Bachelor of Business Administration, Master of Counseling and completion of a one-year research fellowship at Columbia University

Retirement – Sacred Or Scared is the first in a series on retirement escapades. Next one is titled *What The Heck Is A Flume?*

Breinigsville, PA USA
21 September 2009
224462BV00002B/2/P